CW00972123

# Bioethics and the Future of Stem Cell Research

Despite years of heated social controversy over the use of human embryos in embryonic stem cell research, the caravan of stem cell science continues to proceed at an unrelenting pace all around the world. *Bioethics and the Future of Stem Cell Research* urges readers to look beyond the embryo debate to a much wider array of ethical issues in basic stem cell science and clinical translational research, including research involving adult and induced pluripotent stem cells. Insoo Hyun offers valuable insights into complex ethical issues ranging from preclinical animal studies to clinical trials and stem cell tourism, all presented through a unique blend of philosophy, literature, and the history of science, as well as with Dr. Hyun's extensive practical experiences in international stem cell policy formation. This thoughtful book is an indispensible resource for anyone interested in the science of stem cells and the practical and philosophical elements of research ethics.

Insoo Hyun is Associate Professor of Bioethics and Philosophy at Case Western Reserve University School of Medicine. He is an internationally recognized authority on stem cell research ethics. In 2006, he chaired the Subcommittee on Human Biological Materials Procurement for the International Embryonic Stem Cell Guidelines Task Force, a multinational, multidisciplinary working group for the International Society for Stem Cell Research (ISSCR). In 2007, he served as Co-Chairperson of the ISSCR Task Force on International Guidelines for the Clinical Translation of Stem Cells. He is also the past Chairperson of the ISSCR Ethics and Public Policy Committee. His bioethics articles have appeared in *Science, Nature, Cell Stem Cell,* the *Journal of Clinical Investigation,* the *Hastings Center Report,* and the *Cambridge Quarterly of Healthcare Ethics,* among many other publications.

# Bioethics and the Future of Stem Cell Research

INSOO HYUN

*Case Western Reserve University*

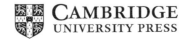

CAMBRIDGE UNIVERSITY PRESS
Cambridge, New York, Melbourne, Madrid, Cape Town,
Singapore, São Paulo, Delhi, Mexico City

Cambridge University Press
32 Avenue of the Americas, New York, NY 10013-2473, USA

www.cambridge.org
Information on this title: www.cambridge.org/9780521127318

First published 2013

Printed in the United States of America

*A catalog record for this publication is available from the British Library.*

*Library of Congress Cataloging in Publication data*
Hyun, Insoo, 1970–
Bioethics and the future of stem cell research / Insoo Hyun.
pages   cm
Includes bibliographical references and index.
ISBN 978-0-521-76869-6 (hardback) – ISBN 978-0-521-12731-8 (paperback)
1. Stem cells – Research – Moral and ethical aspects.   I. Title.
QH588.S83H98   2013
174.2′8–dc23      2012042727

ISBN 978-0-521-76869-6 Hardback
ISBN 978-0-521-12731-8 Paperback

*For my parents,*
*Nak Young Hyun and Moonja Hyun,*
*who supported my study of Philosophy in every way imaginable.*

# Contents

# List of Acronyms

| | |
|---|---|
| ACT | Advanced Cell Technology |
| ASL | American Sign Language |
| CNS | central nervous system |
| DBS | deep brain stimulation |
| DNA | deoxyribonucleic acid |
| EpiSCs | epiblast stem cells |
| ESCRO | Embryonic Stem Cell Research Oversight (Committee) |
| FDA | Food and Drug Administration |
| FGF | fibroblast growth factor |
| GFP | green fluorescent protein |
| GMP | good manufacturing practice |
| GRNOPC1 | Geron's oligodendroglial progenitor cells |
| hES cells | human embryonic stem cells |
| HFEA | Human Fertilisation and Embryology Authority |
| HTA | Human Tissue Authority |
| IACUC | Institutional Animal Care and Use Committee |
| ICU | intensive care unit |
| IND | investigational new drug |
| IOM | Institute of Medicine |
| iPS cells | induced pluripotent stem cells |
| IRB | Institutional Review Board |
| ISSCR | International Society for Stem Cell Research |
| IVF | *in vitro* fertilization |
| JAK | Janus kinase |
| LIF | leukemia inhibitory factor |
| MTA | material transfer agreement |
| NAS | National Academy of Sciences |

| | |
|---|---|
| NIH | National Institutes of Health |
| RAC | Recombinant DNA Advisory Committee |
| RNA | ribonucleic acid |
| SCNT | somatic cell nuclear transfer |
| SCRO | Stem Cell Research Oversight (Committee) |
| STAT | Signal Transducer and Activator of Transcription |

# Acknowledgments

No book is ever the work of a single person. Many individuals have helped inspire my ideas on the ethics of stem cell research, and I wish to acknowledge their influence here. This book has benefited from my informal discussions with many stem cell researchers, clinician-scientists, policy makers, regulators, patient advocates, and philosophers – some of whom are mentioned by name in my chapter footnotes. I am also grateful to my lecture audiences in Beijing, Buenos Aires, Cambridge (UK), Melbourne, and Nijmegen, as well as the Harvard Stem Cell Institute, the Center for iPS Cell Research and Application in Kyoto, the Wallenberg Neuroscience Center at Lund University in Sweden, Singapore General Hospital, Stanford Law School, and the U.S. National Academy of Sciences. Participants and discussants at these meetings helped me sharpen my ideas during the writing of this book.

I am especially grateful to the following individuals who proofread earlier versions of my chapters and provided insightful comments: Carol Gregory, Jonathan Kimmelman, M. William (Willy) Lensch, Patrick L. Taylor, and Paul Tesar. Any deficiencies in this book, conceptual or otherwise, are my own.

Four of my chapters contain portions of articles I published elsewhere. Some elements of Chapter 2 appeared previously in *Cell Stem Cell* (Hyun et al. 2007) and the *Stanford Journal of Law, Science & Policy* (Hyun et al. 2010). A brief portion of Chapter 4 was published in *Clinical Pharmacology and Therapeutics* (Hyun 2011a). A small part of Chapter 5 first appeared in *Cell Stem Cell* (Hyun et al. 2007). And parts of Chapter 8 previously appeared in *Science* (Lindvall and Hyun 2009) and the *Journal of Law, Medicine & Ethics* (Hyun 2010). I thank the editors of these journals for allowing me to include portions of these published articles in this book.

My exploration of the science and ethics of stem cell research began with a faculty research award given to me in 2005 by the Korean-American Educational (Fulbright) Commission and the Fulbright Scholarship Board in Washington, D.C. Their generous financial support allowed me to bridge my interests in philosophy and science in a very concrete manner. My interest in stem cell research ethics was further developed through my service on various committees for the International Society for Stem Cell Research (ISSCR). I thank the ISSCR leadership for giving me the opportunity to work in the area of international stem cell policy formation. This acknowledgment does not imply, however, that the ISSCR leadership necessarily agrees with all of my ideas espoused in this book.

I would also like to thank my mentors over the years, Dan W. Brock, John Ladd, Michael Pritchard, and Stuart Youngner, for encouraging me to pursue a blend of philosophical and professional ethics in my own scholarly research – an approach that should be fully evident to any reader of this book. This book was completed while I was a visiting Erasmus Mundus scholar at Radboud University Nijmegen Medical Center, Nijmegen, the Netherlands. I am grateful to Professor Evert van Leeuwen for sponsoring my visit and for granting me the time and space to finish my manuscript.

Finally, I would like to thank my wife, Leneigh, and my children, Dylan and Morgan, whose love, patience, and support helped make my writing this book possible.

Insoo Hyun
Cleveland, Ohio

# 1

# Prologue

## *The Dogs Bark but the Caravan Moves On*

The Arab proverb in the chapter title offers a concise yet profound statement on the current state of stem cell research.[1] Despite many years of heated social and religious debates over the use of human embryos in embryonic stem cell research, it remains an undeniable fact that the caravan of stem cell science is proceeding at an unrelenting pace around the world. This situation is fascinating in and of itself. On one interpretation, the proverb may represent a fatalistic stance toward stem cell research, where progress in this direction is nothing but an inevitable stage within a naturally unfolding history of science.[2] Or one may interpret it as suggesting the opposite point: that people's economic interests have driven permissive social and scientific ideologies that feed and are conducive to those very same interests.[3]

There is a grain of truth in each of these extreme views. In spite of much controversy, stem cell research continues to advance for several reasons. First, the term *stem cell research* encompasses a very wide range of scientific activity related to many different cell types: multipotent (adult) stem cells; embryonic stem cells and their direct derivatives; and somatic (body) cells that have been bioengineered to take on the pluripotent properties of embryonic stem cells – that is, their capacity to become any

---

[1] This proverb appears in Marcel Proust's *Remembrance of Things Past*, vol. 1 (1913, 497).

[2] This position echoes a Hegelian view of history as the unfolding of universal Reason through the actions of men: "What is actual becomes rational, and the rational becomes actual" (Hegel 1821, 390).

[3] This position is characteristic of Hegel's iconoclast, Marx. "Morality, religion, metaphysics, all the rest of ideology and their corresponding forms of consciousness thus no longer retain the semblance of independence. They have no history, no development; but men, developing their material production and their material intercourse, alter, along with this their real existence, their thinking and the products of their thinking." (Marx 1845, 154–5).

type of cell in the human body.[4] Thus the caravan of stem cell science is composed of many parts and, as I argue in Chapter 2, it must progress together as a whole. Second, stem cell science – especially pluripotent stem cell research – has proven to be of high scientific interest, unfolding previously inaccessible mysteries about human development, genetics, degenerative diseases, and tissue regeneration. As a consequence, groundbreaking discoveries in pluripotent stem cell research have motivated attempts to translate basic stem cell knowledge into practical applications for targeted drug development, new diagnostics, and novel therapeutics for patients with intractable medical conditions – the aims of which carry considerable potential commercial appeal. Without its significant intrinsic and instrumental scientific value, stem cell research would never have garnered legions of support from politicians and policy makers, scientists, and patient advocates; neither could it have ever received such large amounts of public and private funding at all levels: state, national, and international. However, institutional and government support for stem cell research has also driven the need to articulate stem cell–specific regulatory structures to provide social boundaries around stem cell science and, in so doing, facilitate its progress. Thus, multiple interpretations of the Arab proverb are possible as it pertains to stem cell research, and each of these interpretations seems plausible.

In this prologue, I explain the overall approach of this book and introduce its two major themes.[5] I will not rehearse the embryo debate that has dominated stem cell ethics for the past decade. Although the embryo debate is interesting for religious and philosophical reasons, there are major opportunity costs to focusing on just this aspect of the ethical discourse over stem cell research. It is time to move beyond the embryo to a much wider array of ethical issues in basic stem cell science and clinical translational research in which there are potential ethical costs to individuals whom everyone would agree are full moral persons with rights and interests. Both sides of the embryo debate must pay close attention to where the caravan is going and the factors that might influence its direction and speed.

There are those who would argue that one cannot fully appreciate the depth of controversy surrounding the stem cell field unless one begins with the abortion debate sparked by *Roe v. Wade* in 1973 and the

---

4  I explain all of these terms in detail in Chapter 2.
5  Throughout this book I follow the academic philosopher's convention of using the terms *ethical* and *moral* synonymously.

uproar over fetal tissue research in the 1980s, both of which preceded and impacted the development of policies around human embryonic stem (hES) cell research. However, these are characteristically American political-cultural scars, and retracing these old wounds will do little to illuminate the reasons why stem cell research as a whole continues to be ethically sensitive in countries with much more liberal social attitudes toward abortion. To truly understand the origins of the ethical sensitivities of stem cell research within the United States and abroad, one must go back a great deal further to the postmedieval rise of modernity and the emergence and impact of science beginning in the seventeenth century.

Why, some may ask, is it necessary to situate the ethics of stem cell research against the background of these much more expansive historical contexts? I believe many of the deep ethical controversies surrounding most forms of stem cell research today are recapitulations of broader social uncertainties generated by major scientific advancements. Many current ethical disputes in stem cell research appear to be echoes of a familiar clash between two different mind-sets: a premodern faith in a natural world order and a modern enthusiasm for scientific creativity. From its beginnings in the seventeenth century, science has had the capacity to evoke wonder and unease simultaneously. The field of bioethics has emerged in the past several decades as a way to cope with the social tensions caused by science. Because this book is about bioethics about as much as it is about stem cell research, it is appropriate that we set the right contextual tone by retracing the major trains of thought that have influenced the stem cell field and the ethical frameworks of contemporary bioethics. Thus this chapter is meant to serve as a prologue in the most traditional sense of the term. I offer in the next section a background discussion of the scientific worldview that is implicit in all stem cell research. Understanding this embedded *Weltanschauung* is crucial if we want to appreciate the roots of many stem cell controversies today. After discussing the intellectual connections between modern science and the ethics of modernity, I explain in later sections how secular bioethics attempt to provide a means for dealing with the social impacts of stem cell and other scientific advancements.

## The Rise of Science and the Ethics of Modernity

The foundations of modern science were laid in the early seventeenth century when Johannes Kepler (1571–1630) and Galileo Galilei

(1564–1642) confirmed and advanced the astronomical revolution begun by Copernicus some fifty years earlier (Westfall 1999). Later, Isaac Newton (1642–1727) developed the path set forth by his predecessors with his breathtaking systemization of astronomy and dynamics, which permanently removed all traces of Aristotelian animism from the physical world.[6] According to the Newtonian worldview, matter was essentially lifeless and subject only to external causes that were material. The solar system, once having been spun into motion by God, had no further technically explanatory need for His divine intervention. Although modern quantum theory has rejected large swaths of Newtonian physics, it is important to recall just how deeply the scientific revolution represented a rejection of all major currents of medieval thought. Modern quantum theory has done nothing but harden this ideological repudiation.

The seventeenth century was also a time of extraordinary advances beyond astronomy. Improved tools for scientific observation permitted not only more precise viewings of the starry heavens through the telescope, but also extensive explorations of the microscopic world through the compound microscope. Before long the Newtonian Man found himself occupying an uncertain place somewhere between the cold, vast, clockwork universe above and a previously unseen microenvironment oblivious to the gaze of human eyes below.

New scientific observations continued to belie the long-held view of the Middle Ages that all things had a divine purpose involving mankind. Now everything, including the human body, could be understood without the need for religious metaphysics. William Harvey (1578–1657) discovered the closed-circuitry of blood circulation, which he described in terms conducive to a mechanical biology further elaborated by René Descartes in his *Discourse on the Method*.[7] Robert Hooke (1635–1703) observed a piece of cork under a microscope and saw that it was composed of veinlike channels and pores. Hooke was the first to use the biological term *cell* to describe these intricate structures (Westfall 1999). Later, the "Father of Microbiology," Anthony van Leeuwenhoek (1632–1723),

---

[6] Newton was also greatly influenced by Muslim physical theorists who developed many similar ideas of dynamics during the Islamic Golden Age of the eighth to sixteenth centuries. My use of the caravan metaphor is meant to allude in part to the connection between the Western scientific revolution and the Middle East.

[7] The full title of Descartes's work is *Discourse on the Method of Rightly Conducting One's Reason and Seeking the Truth in the Sciences* (1637). Historians of science widely acknowledge this as the first popular comprehensive articulation of the scientific method. Writing in French rather than Latin, Descartes intended to aim his anti-Aristotelian treatise to a broad, nonacademic audience.

used his improvements on the microscope to observe spermatozoa and to discover unicellular organisms. No one at the time conceived of the possibility that Leeuwenhoek's tiny organisms bore any relation to the cells that Hooke found in plants. It was not until twentieth-century molecular genetics, built on the foundations laid by Darwin and Mendel, that the apparent heterogeneity of nature could be explained using the common language of DNA, not divine creation.

With the steady rise of scientific belief systems in the seventeenth century came a corresponding decline in ecclesiastical authority (Russell 1945). Although early scientists such as Newton and his intellectual cohorts were pious men, their activities were profoundly disconcerting to the religious orthodoxy. In addition to the truism that Man was ousted from the center of the heliocentric universe, the scientific revolution signaled a radical shift in what thoughtful persons were willing to accept as the justificatory grounds for their beliefs. The authority of science revealed itself to be a very different creature from the authority of the Church, as the former was intellectual and evidence based, while the latter was authoritative and faith based. Unlike medieval religious dogma, which laid down a complete system of beliefs that was accepted as indubitable and incorrigible, science offered piecemeal and tentative conclusions that were always subject to doubt and modification. While medieval dogmatists were persons of unshakeable faith, even in the face of countervailing facts, the scientific mind was skeptical and called for probabilistic evidence.

One should not conclude, however, that the scientific mind-set left its adherents feeling completely helpless. Rapid advances in the theoretical and practical sciences, while humbling to mankind's position in the universe, had the cumulative effect of imparting a notion that one could exert greater human control over the physical world. This newfound sense of scientific power in the seventeenth century was met with the arrival of early liberal individualism as characterized by the political philosophy of John Locke (1632–1704) and others who promoted the ideals of enlightened self-interest and conditional governmental authority.[8]

---

[8] Locke, *Second Treatise of Government* (1690). Locke argued in his second treatise that civil government was based on a social contract and not something established by divine authority. The *raison d'être* of government was the mutual advantage of men, especially with respect to the protection of their private property interests. Locke wrote his second treatise while operating with a group of conspirators led by the first Earl of Shaftesbury to resist the sovereign. Locke's work provided the theoretical justification for the Whig Revolution and the installation of William and Mary in 1689.

The ideological movement of philosophical liberalism valued property rights, commerce, industry, and democracy. It was, at heart, a brand of political and ethical antiauthoritarianism that stressed the importance of self-governance, individual rights, liberty, and reason – values that resonated harmoniously with the scientific ethos of the nascent modern era.[9] Like the physical world, long-standing social and political institutions and traditions also came to be viewed as malleable according to the dictates of human rational power.

The emerging ethics of modernity stood in sharp contrast to the natural law tradition of medievalists like St. Thomas Aquinas (1226–74). According to Aquinas and the scholastic moral theologians of the Middle Ages, God was the giver of the natural law through His divine providence and in accordance with His eternal plan (Aquinas 1274). Mankind is able to understand the precepts of natural law through reason and act freely on them. The precepts of natural law directed all rational beings to pursue their good as God had planned.

Within Aquinas's paradigmatic natural law theory one can detect two crucial differences that separate the medieval natural law tradition from the ethics of modernity. First, because the precepts of natural law are an aspect of divine providence, it is possible for an action to be morally wrong regardless of whether individuals freely consent to it or whether the act produces no appreciable harms to the parties involved. Actions can be wrong simply by virtue of being "unnatural" as determined by God's wisdom and grace. According to the ethics of modernity, however, the moral worth of human actions was to be determined by the voluntary and rational autonomy interests of individuals and/or the balance of measurable harms and benefits produced. In the moral judgment of the moderns, then, it would be conceptually incoherent to assert that an action or state of affairs could be wrong if no rights were violated and no physical or psychological harms were suffered. In the absence of either source of wrongfulness, an action would have to be judged purely on prudential, aesthetic, or perfectionist grounds.

Second, God's existence was absolutely necessary for the medieval natural law tradition because it was God's divine plan that gave the precepts

---

[9] This harmony was no mere coincidence. Locke studied philosophy and medicine at Oxford, and his scientific talents led to his election to the prestigious Royal Society in 1668. At Oxford he was mentored by the mechanical philosopher Robert Boyle, who, with the help of his assistant Robert Hooke, built an air pump that led to the formulation of Boyle's law. Thus the easy convergence of science and the ethics of modernity should come as no surprise, because Locke's social philosophies and epistemology sprang from a mind trained to think scientifically.

of natural law their normative force.[10] God, while present in the minds of many early modern ethical theorists, was not philosophically necessary in order to make modern ethical theories internally consistent and plausible. Unlike medieval ethics, the ethics of modernity was focused around rational self-governance and the psychological/behavioral inclinations of all human beings.[11] Like the god of Newton's universe, the god of modern ethical systems could be viewed as having little else to do outside of imbuing human beings with reason and the passions and leaving them to rule themselves. This shift toward conceptualizing ethical standards in terms of rational human behavior marked a new surge in secular ethical thinking, one that still characterizes most academic moral philosophy today.

Thus the seventeenth century was bookended by the emergence of scientific thinking and the development of modern philosophical thought. Between these two epochal intellectual movements lay the old scholastic worldview of the medievalists slowly losing its grip of influence. The dogs barked but the caravan of modernity moved on. The strict exclusion of psychic forces from physical nature and the consequent theoretical dispensability of God from modern moral philosophy were among two of the most important legacies of seventeenth-century thought.

## Power and Uncertainty

However, the intellectual legacies of early modernity had to be purchased at the price of people's sense of security in their epistemic beliefs and moral judgments. We still bear the weight of these intellectual costs several centuries later, even in our thinking about stem cell research. Like the Newtonian Man who found himself occupying an uncertain place between the vast universe above and the microenvironment below, modernists today find themselves on a lifeboat with very few permanently fixed planks. To their right are the premodern faithful still operating

---

[10] There are nontheistic natural law theorists, e.g., Philippa Foot (2001), who ground the precepts of natural law in a vaguely Aristotelian conception of human flourishing. It bears pointing out, however, that nontheistic natural law theories are consistent with what I am calling here *modern secular ethical theories*, because being avoidably prevented from full human flourishing counts as a type of harm and is thus morally wrong from a modernist's point of view.

[11] Each of these approaches was epitomized in the eighteenth century by the moral philosophies of Immanuel Kant and the utilitarians. Although utilitarianism has never been a theistic moral doctrine, Kantianism and neo-Kantianism today are usually treated as secular theories.

under a natural law tradition that frames all scientific and social issues under the lens of a theistic worldview. To their left are the postmodern relativists who doubt whether any moral and scientific conclusions have objective authority beyond a tribal circle of like-minded cultural players.[12]

Besides warding off philosophical attacks from both sides, the modernists must also negotiate a host of indeterminacies within the ethics of modernity. Modern ethical theories tend to define morally right actions in one of two ways: either an action is right because it corresponds to people's moral rights and duties (deontological ethical theories) or because it produces the greatest balance of benefits over harms for those affected (consequentialist ethical theories). Although each of these ethical approaches has the advantage of providing a common moral language within modern pluralistic societies, they also leave plenty of unanswered questions.

First is the issue of how these two approaches relate to one another, because consequentialism and deontology offer a plausible account of morally right actions, so plausible that modern ethicists often shift from one approach to the other when deliberating over complex ethical issues. On one view of this interactivity, people's rights constitute a moral floor below which consequentialist ethical justifications must never dip. To put the point another way, rights trump considerations of overall ethical utility (Dworkin 1978). For example, it would not be morally acceptable to credit a famous scientist for an important discovery made by his student even if doing so would greatly elevate its acceptance and scientific impact. The student has a basic right to be treated fairly and not have her work plagiarized. According to another view, however, it is consequentialism that sets a moral ceiling on the deontological approach by limiting the extent of people's rights. On this view, rights are not absolute in the sense that they must be respected in all circumstances. This limit-setting approach finds its most well-known articulation in John Stuart Mill's Harm-to-Others Principle, which maintains that personal liberties should

---

[12] For a comprehensive critique of all varieties of relativism see Allen Wood (2002). Philosophical postmodernists may criticize my analysis in this chapter by questioning my implicit acceptance of modern concepts such as ethical justification and scientific and historical knowledge. I will not engage in a debate here about the merits of postmodern modes of thought. Jürgen Habermas (1987) has advanced a scathing critique of philosophical postmodernism whereby he argues that postmodernist arguments characteristically presuppose the very concepts they seek to undermine and in that way are guilty of a performative contradiction.

be respected to the point at which their exercise would lead to serious harms to identifiable individuals (Mill 1859). For instance, patients have a right to refuse medical interventions, unless they suffer from highly infectious diseases that pose a grave and immediate public health threat to others. Deontological and consequentialist moral views cannot stand completely in isolation from one another, for people's rights and the overall good matter in our everyday moral judgments. But rights often come into conflict with efforts to promote the greatest total benefits, and it remains an open question as to which of these two ethical approaches ought to set limits on the other.

Second, there are serious philosophical indeterminacies within each of these modern ethical approaches. For example, deontologists must offer an account of how to balance conflicts among people's rights. When two or more rights clash (as they so often do in difficult moral dilemmas) how does one determine which of these rights is more "fundamental" and thus should take precedence? Consequentialists, too, must struggle with ambiguities. For instance, a proposed action may produce large benefits in the near term but far fewer benefits later, while an alternative choice may produce fewer benefits now but greater benefits in the future. How far into the horizon of future possibilities should a consequentialist look in determining the moral worth of a specified act? Furthermore, how is she supposed to decide which of her proposed alternatives is most likely to have its believed effects, good and bad? How should one compare different possible outcomes, especially when they relate to different domains of value?[13] And how should the consequentialist demarcate the relevant circle of individuals affected by each alternative choice? Given these and other indeterminacies, the real-world impacts of a consequentialist's ethical choices can be notoriously difficult to prognosticate.[14] All of these indeterminacies will come into play when we examine the various ethical controversies concerning stem cell research.

---

[13] I explore this particular problem, which I call the *incommensurability problem*, in greater detail in Chapter 7.

[14] It should be pointed out that, on a consequentialist moral approach, it is not enough simply to believe that an action is likely to produce beneficial effects. Technically, according to consequentialism, an action cannot be determined to be right or wrong until its effects have actually been produced; thus in all cases the consequentialist must attach the moral value of an action retrospectively. This is a counterintuitive account of our everyday moral judgments, because most people believe that actions are either right or wrong at the time in which they are performed, not that actions must be determined to be right or wrong in hindsight, as consequentialism requires.

These uncertainties embedded in secular ethics should come as no surprise, because uncertainty has proven to be one of the key defining characteristics of modernity. The modern world, built on the seemingly unshakable foundations of science and enlightened rationality, has turned out to be a surprisingly unpredictable realm. Geological disturbances of thought triggered by scientific advances at the bedrock continue to unsettle the inhabitants of the modern age. Periodic seismic shifts in what persons took for granted as the *terra firma* of their beliefs have provoked a desire among many to return to a premodern view in which our tilting world can be righted by the steady hand of a beneficent god. United by their common anxiety, some theists and nontheists have joined in the call to halt scientific activities deemed to be "unnatural" and fundamentally destabilizing. In contrast, the response of the moderns has been to embrace the redemptive uses of their newfound scientific powers, thus rechanneling the seismic impacts of science into a protective armor to defend mankind's vulnerabilities. This capacity of science to evoke fear and wonder simultaneously, to unsettle and empower, has always been an ineliminable element of modernity. So it is within the context of these dueling forces originating in the seventeenth century – power and uncertainty – that the science and ethics of stem cell research must be analyzed.

## Stem Cell Research: New Science and Old Tensions

Stem cell science is ethically controversial for many of the same reasons that make other paradigm-shifting science controversial. All forms of controversial science tend to disrupt the categories we use to organize the world around us. Stem cell research has taught us in very short order that our long-standing beliefs about human development and biological potentiality must be revised. Biologists had held for centuries that the developmental process by which a single cell (zygote) becomes a complete human being was a one-way street. The primitive stem cells of the developing embryo were thought to differentiate down different pathways to form specialized cells that remain in their specialized state until the day they die. But now stem cell science is teaching us how to control and even reverse this developmental process. We are learning that all of our specialized cells are malleable and can be transformed into any other cell type (see Chapter 2). Stem cell science has repaved the developmental process into a two-way street where scientists can direct cells to travel from a stem cell state to a specialized state and vice versa. We are now in the process of learning how to bend biological development and tissue formation to our will; human cells are increasingly becoming viewed as plastic biological materials to be shaped according to our own practical purposes. The true power of stem cell research may lie in the ability to determine what our cells will do.

Stem cell research is also forcing us to revise our views about biological potentiality. Aristotelian potentiality, the view of the premoderns, held that biological development was the actualization of an intrinsic power, an inner striving, of a budding organism to grow into what it was meant to be. But advances in stem cell science have shown that biological potentiality is far more a matter of personal and social choice than previously conceived (Testa 2009). For instance, under the right technical conditions, and given a series of collective choices, each of our body cells has the potential to generate a whole new human life (Hyun 2008).

It should be acknowledged that "potentiality" has been under revision for several decades, and stem cell research is merely applying the latest touches on this revisionary process. It was the *in vitro* (in a dish) fertilization (IVF) revolution of the late 1970s that first alerted the public to the view that biological potentiality could be largely subject to human choice. It was shown then that, given our ability to combine sperm and egg outside a woman's body and thereby select what to do with the resulting zygotes, even the earliest stages of human reproduction could be manipulated. The potential for fertility clinic embryos to develop into complete human beings hinged crucially on people's choices regarding whether they would be transferred to a woman's uterus or used for some other purpose. This power to determine the fate of *ex corporeal* embryos, to be able to divorce them from their so-called Aristotelian trajectory toward birth, continues to be deeply unsettling for some, particularly the premodern faithful who believe that every embryo has a predetermined purpose for life. According to the analysis I am proposing here, the ongoing embryo debate in stem cell research is actually a symptom of a broader social discomfort caused by this widening of human developmental potentiality to include a far greater element of personal choice and control. In my view, the stem cell controversy is driven by concerns far wider than merely the embryo debate.

Stem cell science is transformative and disruptive. As the history of science has repeatedly shown, the possibility that anything can be suddenly upended prompts a wish among many to demarcate clearly how things ought to remain, be it according to a natural law tradition or some other preestablished normative worldview. But these instinctive responses all miss a crucial point – namely, that it is the so-called stable, traditional categories that are constantly being put into crisis by science. Power, uncertainty, choice, and unease are all inescapable aspects of modernity. The dogs bark but the caravan of stem cell science moves on. What should we do in light of this fact, when our old concepts no longer provide the shelter we seek? To critically engage this question is the stuff of bioethics.

## What Is Bioethics?

Not all readers may be familiar with bioethics as a secular academic discipline, or how it relates to the various themes covered in this chapter. Secular bioethics must be understood first and foremost as a direct outgrowth of modernity.[15] It has developed over the past several decades as a means to cope with the moral and philosophical ambiguities driven by rapid scientific and technological advances in the life sciences (Callahan 2003).

Bioethics first arose in the United States in the 1960s under circumstances reminiscent of the forces that propelled seventeenth-century thought. It was born at the crux of three extraordinary social developments: the antitraditionalism and personal liberationism of the civil rights and feminist movements, and the antiauthoritarian political ethos ignited by the Vietnam War. During this era of rapid social change, with its heavy emphasis on the modern ideals of personal independence and choice, came also a swift expansion of advanced medical technologies. New generations of patients rebelled against the ancient Hippocratic tradition of medical paternalism and insisted that they, not their doctors, should be the final determiners of their own medical treatment. And the choices they faced were tough and nearly endless. The 1960s underscored a dramatic shift in how health care was delivered in the United States and other industrialized countries. New technological breakthroughs were coupled with decades-old advances in public health, thus transforming more rapidly the epidemiology of the death experience. Death, which was once usually suffered at home under the shroud

---

[15] I acknowledge that the early days of bioethics were also strongly influenced by Catholic moral theology. However, I focus my discussion in this chapter and in this book on the secular bioethics tradition, which owes much of its roots to modern moral philosophy and the norms of secular professional ethics. There are other accounts of the origins of American bioethics that are slightly different from mine which the reader should consult, such as Albert Jonsen's *The Birth of Bioethics* (1998) and David Rothman's *Strangers at the Bedside* (1991).

of an infectious disease, now became a much more publically visible event in a hospital at the long end of a protracted, degenerative disease. The 1960s were marked by the introduction of many advanced medical interventions, such as kidney dialysis, organ transplantation, intensive care units (ICUs), and mechanical ventilators. With the use of these and other advanced medical technologies, a patient's process of dying became something that could be drawn out and controlled, something that could be decided upon by the patient or surrogates regarding the rate at which the patient would be allowed to slide to the bottom of a downward slope. The old adage of simply letting nature "take its course" was no longer accepted as the default ethical position for all end-of-life cases.

But, as the familiar refrain goes, with increases in medical power and choice came the corresponding haze of uncertainty. Advances in medical technology threw people's previously stable categories into disarray. For instance, when hospital ICUs developed the capacity to sustain severely brain-damaged patients on mechanical ventilators, new philosophical questions quickly arose. According to the traditional criterion for determining death – the cessation of heart and lung function – ICU patients under these circumstances qualified as being alive so long as they remained on ventilator support. But physicians and families began to wonder whether some severely brain-damaged patients had already died in some morally relevant sense and whether the machines were left "doing all the work." Were all of these patients alive in a philosophical sense, which would call into action the usual moral duties of the physician, or were some patients merely breathing cadavers? This was not purely a medical or legal matter, for medicine and the law could offer little guidance; it was at heart an ethical dilemma that called for a new method of determining death. The old concept of what it meant to be dead had to be revised. In due course, the whole-brain criterion that developed directly out of this ethical challenge led to the seemingly counterintuitive conclusion that some ICU patients could be considered dead even though they continued to breathe and their hearts continued to beat.

Ever since the early days of bioethics in the 1960s, society has continued to have difficulty assimilating new scientific and technological changes, especially when these changes challenge people's preexisting categories. These struggles have driven an ongoing need for bioethical inquiry. Today bioethics is a thriving field in its own right, as an academic discipline and as a social force of some consequence in medicine, biomedical research, public health, and public policy (Callahan 2003). Despite the enormous breadth of bioethics, which ranges from interpersonal conflicts in medical practice, to ethical issues in animal and human subjects research, to policy formation in health care and the sciences, the bioethics field may be united by two common characteristics.

First, bioethics is by nature a highly interdisciplinary activity. As vexing ethical issues in health care and the life sciences began to arise, it soon became apparent that these extraordinarily complex problems would have to be addressed from multiple points of view, be it philosophy, law, medicine, or the social and biological sciences. For example, it has become widely acknowledged that bioethics in the clinic requires moral decision makers to begin by taking seriously the trade-offs of different medical alternatives to patients and the everyday realities of how health care is delivered. Likewise, the bioethics of research must begin (as I emphasize in later chapters) with a firm grasp of the science involved and a careful consideration of the ongoing scientific narrative of discovery that a particular research project aims to address.

Second, bioethics tends to be practiced today along the main modalities of the ethics of modernity. That is, the predominant forms of ethical reasoning in secular bioethics are consequentialism and deontology, broadly construed.[16] In pluralistic modern societies, these two varieties of secular ethical thought have been conducive to sorting through bioethical dilemmas facing individuals who do not share the same cultural and religious traditions. By appealing to what may be called "commonly accessible" ethical reasons (e.g., rights and harms), contemporary bioethicists strive to frame bioethical issues and arguments in terms that are understandable and persuasive to persons of different faiths and personal belief systems. The secular approach of bioethics today may be further explained by the fact that bioethics on the whole tend to thrive in societies that have rapid technological advancements as well as democratic political systems that afford persons the liberty to make up their own minds regarding matters of faith and their own personal ideological commitments. That bioethics is an outgrowth of modernity is not an overstatement.

However, as an aspect of the ethics of modernity, bioethics has inherited all the previously mentioned indeterminacies plaguing the secular ethics of rights, duties, and consequences. How are difficult bioethical dilemmas supposed to be resolved in pluralistic modern societies when it is unclear from the start what the limitations of people's rights-claims are

---

[16] Virtue ethics and others still fit under these categories, in the most general sense.

and what the proper informational inputs ought to be for consequential-ist moral frameworks? Bioethics raises plenty of difficult questions, much as the ethics of modernity did on a broader scale. Who should control emerging technologies? What kinds of regulations are needed to con-trol the steady tide of new biomedical advances? Should the benefits of new scientific and medical advances be broadly distributed? Bioethical inquiry involves technology-driven dilemmas facing individuals, institu-tions, and societies all living under a common cloud of uncertainty – uncertainty over how best to balance harms and benefits, about our obligations to others, and about the extent to which we ought to exercise our newfound powers.

## The Chimera Myth and Two Major Themes

This book deals with pressing research ethics issues in stem cell science (and, to a lesser extent, clinical ethics as it pertains to the use of new stem cell–based therapies). Research ethics is a subarea of bioethics that addresses the moral aims and conduct of scientific investigation. Research ethics is, in my view, the chief means by which modern societies attempt to manage the potentially harmful effects of scientific inquiry. The Greek myth of the Chimera can be used to illustrate this key point – that transformative technologies require ongoing ethical control, and I shall refer to this myth to introduce the two main themes of this book.

Human/nonhuman chimera studies have emerged as one of the most heated postembryo controversies in stem cell research. Human/nonhu-man chimeras are created when human stem cells or their derivatives are transferred into animal hosts during the course of basic and pre-clinical stem cell research. Some commentators have argued that this type of research should not be performed on grounds that it is wrong to blur the line between humans and other animal species by mixing significant levels of human biological materials into laboratory animals (Robert and Baylis 2003). Premodernists may point to the origin of the word *chimera* – the terrible fire-breathing Greek monster that was part lion, part goat, and part serpent – as suggestive of the wrongfulness of chimera research (see Figure 1.1). Some might argue that the original Chimera was a horrible aberration, and that stem cell–based chimeras are just as abominable and a threat to the natural order.

But I would argue that a closer consideration of the Chimera myth reveals a very different moral message. The Chimera was eventu-ally defeated by the Greek mortal Bellerophon (Hamilton 1942).

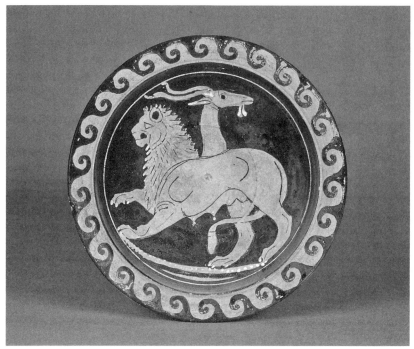

FIGURE 1.1. The Greek Chimera.
Credit: © RMN-Grand Palais/Art Resource, NY. Description: Red Figure Plate:
Chimera. 3rd quarter 4th century BCE. K362. Photo: Hervé Lewandowski.
Location: Louvre (Museum), Paris, France.

Athena, the goddess of wisdom, descended from Mount Olympus and gave Bellerophon a golden bridle, which he used to tame Pegasus. Interestingly, Pegasus was also a chimeric animal – a winged horse – but was an admired mythic creature among the Greeks. Using the golden bridle, Bellerophon rode Pegasus and killed the Chimera from on high with a quiver full of arrows (see Figure 1.2).

Bellerophon and Pegasus went on to have several more adventures together, defeating many Greek enemies. Eventually, Bellerophon became so successful that he decided he too was a god and tried to ride Pegasus to Mount Olympus to take his place next to the other Greek deities. Pegasus rebelled and threw Bellerophon off his back. Bellerophon spent the rest of his days crippled and blind (Hamilton 1942). The lesson to be drawn from the Chimera story, if one examines the myth from beginning to end, is that it is not the chimerism of an animal per se that gives it its moral worth, but rather how the chimeric animal is used and what role it plays in society. The Chimera myth is

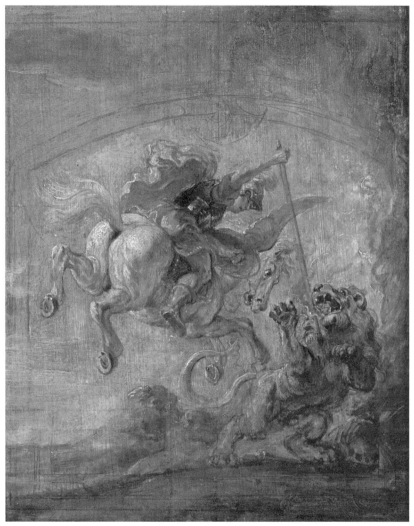

FIGURE 1.2. Bellerophon and Pegasus battle the Chimera.
Credit: © RMN-Grand Palais/Art Resource, NY. Description: Bellerophon on
Pegasus piercing the Chimera with a lance. Oil sketch on wood, 34 × 27.5 cm.
Inv.: 458. Photo: René-Gabriel Ojéda. Artist: Rubens, Peter Paul (1577–1640).
Location: Musee Bonnat, Bayonne, France.

ultimately a warning about hubris and the use of transformative technology for selfish ends.

My approach to analyzing the Chimera myth is indicative of my overall approach to stem cell research ethics – context matters. For the purposes of this book, context matters in three important senses.

First, in order to determine the moral worth of an action, one must look at the full context of the subject at hand. For example, merely pointing to the horror of the Chimera and suggesting that human-to-animal stem cell chimeras are equally objectionable is to take the Chimera myth out of context. In matters of ethics, it is not enough to examine simply what philosophers call the "intrinsic properties" of a person or thing; one must also pay attention to what are called its "relational properties" – that is, how that thing relates to or interacts with aspects of the world around it.

Second, in assessing the ethical permissibility of a stem cell study proposal, be it an animal study or a human clinical trial, one must place the study proposal in its proper context. That is, the research proposal must constitute a step forward in an ongoing scientific narrative, in which it must connect justifiably to earlier experiments and contribute to knowledge of the history of the problem under study. In the ethical review of stem cell research, then, context also matters. One cannot adequately judge the ethical permissibility of a stem cell study in isolation from its broader scientific context.

Third, context matters in a biological sense for stem cells. Human stem cells depend on developmental cues from the microenvironment of the host into which they are placed, be it an animal or a human being. The host's bodily niche environment helps "instruct" the stem cells what to do. So, in this way, biological context matters crucially for stem cell development and stem cell behavior. Opponents of human/nonhuman chimera research and proponents of rapid human clinical trials may not be aware of this interdependent relationship between stem cells and their niche. For instance, opponents of chimera research fear that the transfer of human stem cells into animals may give rise to human psychological and moral characteristics in the resulting chimeric animals. But this worry overlooks the fact that human stem cells do not carry with them a complete human "essence" or Aristotelian "agency" when placed into animals' bodily niche environments. Furthermore, those who would wish to proceed rapidly to stem cell clinical trials must be reminded that stem cells and their derivatives may have very different, unpredictable actions when placed in areas of the body different from the microenvironments in which these stem cells are normally found.

In summary, the first major theme of this book is that, in order to assess the ethics of stem cell research, one must attend to each of these varieties of context: (1) the moral narrative surrounding the action, (2) the scientific narrative surrounding the research project, and (3) the biological context into which the stem cells are transferred.

My use of the Chimera myth also introduces a second major theme of this book. In asking "What makes research ethical?" one can ask this question on either of two levels. At a broadly philosophical, conceptual level, one may ask, "Why is it right to do research? In what ways is research good for society? And what are the central human values at stake?" On a narrower construal of the question, one may ask, "What makes a particular research project ethically permissible? What criteria should be used to mark the difference(s) between an ethical research project and an unethical one?"

I call the first level *philosophical research ethics* and the second level *practical research ethics.* Philosophical research ethics concerns the ethical aims of science and the relationship between science and society. Practical research ethics concerns the practicable regulatory requirements in a local research setting that constitute the institutional criteria for permissible research. The golden bridle at the center of the Chimera myth is a metaphor for both these levels of research ethics. On the one hand, Athena's golden bridle represents philosophical research ethics as the stuff of philosophical wisdom, our rationally directed prudence to control the natural world for the purposes of human flourishing. On the other hand, the golden bridle also represents practical research ethics as the means by which science is controlled and steered at the local level – the modern-day manifestation of Bellerophon's golden bridle that provides hands-on control over the actual conduct of research.

Thus it is another major message of this book that philosophical research ethics and practical research ethics matter crucially in our ethical discourse over stem cells. Traditionally, opponents of stem cell research argue from the broader, philosophical level while proponents, who have already accepted a permissive ideology concerning stem cell research, focus their energies on the practical, regulatory level. Neither side in the stem cell debate actually engages successfully and directly with the other's concerns, for they tend to speak from two different levels. Opponents raise fears about scientific hubris and the devaluing of nascent human life and the natural order, while proponents respond with a series of regulatory proposals, as if practical ethical reinforcements were sufficient to rebut their opponents' concerns at the philosophical level.

Throughout this book I argue that the future of stem cell science is rife with many ethical pitfalls and challenges that could threaten the rights and interests of persons involved in the research, either as human biological materials donors, research subjects, patients, or scientists in the field. Thus it is crucial that we engage now in a sustained analysis of the downstream ethical issues stemming from the current trajectory of human stem cell research. The caravan of stem cell science continues to march on. The instinctive response of opponents to call for a halt to this procession ignores the historical fact that this request has never stopped revolutionary science from seeking the next turn in the road. In contrast to this unease, there is the modern confidence that the disruptive powers of science can be redirected to benefit humanity at large. Whether this confidence is well grounded will depend ultimately on the adequacy of the ethics of modernity. Many will view this link as a blessing and a curse.

# 2

## A Shifting Terrain

### *The Dynamics of Stem Cell Research*

What is the best way to think about stem cell research? What are its unique characteristics, and which of these features are ethically important? Let us address these questions systematically. Stem cell research is first and foremost a scientific discipline. From this obvious point follows a series of important considerations often overlooked in stem cell ethical debates.

First, as a scientific endeavor – with academic linkages dating back to the rise of the modern worldview – stem cell research eschews large swaths of premodern thought, such as Aristotelian animism, in favor of modern materialist explanations. For example, rather than maintaining, as the Aristotelian Scholastics did, that nascent human bodies are impelled to unfold an innate developmental nature through the workings of an animating soul, stem cell scientists embrace the mechanistic view that human biological development is nothing more than a cascade of innumerable physical events.[1] Thus one of the primary goals of stem cell scientists is to understand how the soulless chemistry of genetic information becomes translated into the development of tissues and complex organ systems.

Second, stem cell research exists within an interconnected web of many other scientific disciplines. Arising from the intellectual traditions of cell and developmental biology, stem cell science now intersects with previously separate contemporary fields such as neurology, hematology, cardiology, and gastroenterology, to name a few. Cell and molecular biologists from diverse medical fields are drawn to stem cell research by their common interest in trying to understand how cells, tissues, and organs

---

[1] This point is especially important for our discussion of human/nonhuman chimera research in Chapter 5.

are formed and repaired (Daley 2010). Because it is so deeply embedded within a broad array of scientific areas, it would be impossible to stop stem cell research without negatively impacting numerous other fields in the biological sciences.

Third, as a scientific endeavor in its own right, stem cell research has become an extraordinarily complex and diverse interdisciplinary field. To help organize this broad range of activity, we can categorize stem cell research under two general headings. *Basic stem cell research* addresses fundamental questions about tissue formation and human development, including the developmental course of serious genetic and degenerative diseases. *Translational stem cell research* involves the practical applications of a wide array of stem cell types and their derivatives for drug discovery and the development of new clinical therapies. In order to explore the ethics of stem cell research in a comprehensive manner, we must become familiar with this broad range of scientific activity and the many important interrelations therein.

Each of these considerations impacts how we frame our ethical analyses of stem cell research in the following chapters. Good bioethics must begin with a solid grasp of the object of analysis. Thus, if we wish to discuss the ethics of stem cell research intelligently, we must bear in mind the modern worldview that stem cell science represents, its relationship to other scientific fields, and its technical details and challenges. In this chapter I explain the varieties of basic and clinical translational stem cell research, their interrelationships, and future trends. The stem cell research terrain is constantly shifting, where progress in one area of stem cell research will depend on lessons learned in another area. In surveying this terrain, I shall flag the emerging scientific and ethical issues that accompany current trajectories in basic and translational stem cell research, issues that will be explored at greater length in subsequent chapters.

## Stem Cells as a Scientific and Philosophical Object of Analysis

We begin our inquiry with the age-old philosophical maneuver of defining our object of analysis. What are stem cells? This, we find, is an extraordinarily rich question. Let us start with the simplest answer, and then proceed to a much more nuanced response.

The most basic scientific answer is that stem cells are primitive, undifferentiated cells that have the capacity to make new copies of themselves (self-renew) and to specialize (differentiate) into various other cell types, such as blood, muscle, and nerve cells. Traditionally, stem cells

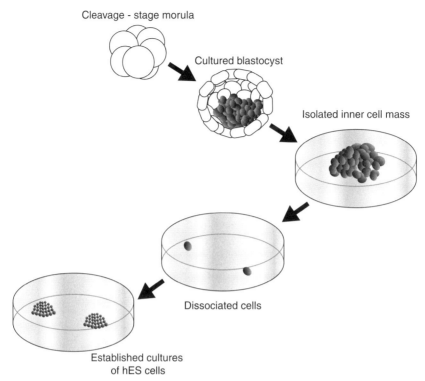

FIGURE 2.1. hES cell derivation.
Artist: Jeffrey T. Siliko.

have been categorized into two main groups: embryonic stem cells and adult stem cells.[2]

Human embryonic stem cells are isolated from five-day-old embryos during the blastocyst stage of early development prior to implantation in the womb (see Figure 2.1).[3] These primitive cells later give rise to all

---

[2] Although adult cell research has existed for more than 40 years and has led to clinical therapies for leukemia and other blood disorders, the field of hES cell research is still relatively new, and basic discoveries have yet to be directly transitioned into clinical applications. Human embryonic stem cells were first isolated and maintained in culture in 1998 by James Thomson and colleagues at the University of Wisconsin. Since then, more than a thousand different isolates of self-renewing hES cells (stem cell lines) have been created and shared by researchers worldwide.

[3] As pointed out in Chapter 1, a key developmental fact often ignored by opponents of hES cell research is that fertility clinic embryos need to be implanted in order to realize fully their biological potential. That is, preimplantation embryos need cues from the maternal body to trigger their next cascade of developmental events. Absent the

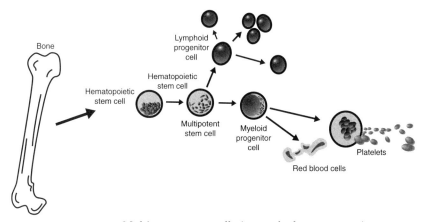

FIGURE 2.2. Multipotent stem cells (example: bone marrow).
Artist: Jeffrey T. Siliko.

the different cells and organ systems of the fetus. Embryonic stem cells are pluripotent because they are capable of differentiating along each of the three germ layers – the ectoderm (e.g., skin, nerves, and brain), the mesoderm (e.g., bone and muscle), and the endoderm (e.g., lungs and digestive system) – in addition to producing the germ line (sperm and eggs).

During later stages of human development, minute quantities of more mature stem cells can be found in most tissue and organ systems, such as bone marrow, the skin, and the gut. These mature stem cells are responsible for renewing and repairing the body's specialized cells (see Figure 2.2).

Although they are often referred to by the lay public as "adult" stem cells, they can be found in fetuses and newborns and in umbilical cord blood. Researchers prefer to call these stem cells multipotent because they are less versatile than pluripotent stem cells. In humans, multipotent stem cells have not been decisively shown to transdifferentiate across different cell lineages without significant laboratory manipulation.[4] Thus most stem cell scientists believe multipotent stem cells are normally

decision to implant fertility clinic embryos, their "potential for full human life" exists in only the most abstract, hypothetical sense. To ignore this simple fact about human development is to accept a false quasi-Aristotelian notion of the embryo's (wholly) innate potentiality.

[4]   Transdifferentiation from one cell lineage to another (mesoderm, ectoderm, and endoderm) is not a "normal" characteristic of multipotent stem cells (George Daley, personal communication).

restricted to differentiating into cells related to the tissue or organ systems from which the multipotent stem cells originated (e.g., blood stem cells into blood cells and muscle stem cells into muscle fibers). Unlike pluripotent stem cells, multipotent stem cells can differentiate into cells representing either just the germ line (i.e., sperm and eggs) or just *one* of the three germ layers (i.e., ectoderm, endoderm, and mesoderm).

Some readers may find these various stem cell terms confusing. It might be helpful therefore to organize the terminology in the following manner. The terms *embryonic* and *adult* signify the origins of the stem cells in question. The terms *pluripotent* and *multipotent* signify the capabilities of stem cells – that is, whether they are able to differentiate into all types of cells or a more limited range. Because these two pairs of terms signify two different aspects of stem cells – where they came from and what they can do – we must not assume that the terms *embryonic* and *adult* can be used synonymously with *pluripotent* and *multipotent.*

Not only do these pairs of terms pick out different aspects of stem cells, but I believe there are also good reasons to employ the capabilities terminology of stem cells over the origins terminology. For one, the language of "embryonic" and "adult" stem cells has become so politically charged that it could obscure some ethical considerations that may be of importance for persons who hold firm, but nuanced, personal views about abortion and stem cell research.

The origins terminology tends to be favored by persons for whom the origin of stem cells deeply matters – for example, antiabortionists and politicians who are opposed to hES cell research. But here we must be careful not to be misled by some of the commonsense connotations of the origins terminology. To a layperson, the terms *adult* and *embryonic* may suggest that (1) adult stem cells are obtained from mature individuals who can offer informed consent for their extraction and scientific use, and that (2) embryonic stem cells are harvested from fetuses following electively terminated pregnancies. (Some foes of embryonic stem cell research seem to have capitalized on these commonsense assumptions.)

However, these lay presumptions do not survive close scrutiny. As I noted previously, all adult stem cells can be found in developing fetuses. Fetuses have been a convenient source of adult stem cells that are difficult to obtain without permanently and gravely harming grown individuals. For example, much neural adult stem cell research has been conducted using stem cells harvested from the central nervous systems (CNSs) of electively aborted fetuses. So, people's attempts to ethically distance adult stem cell research from abortion are misguided.

The supposed direct link between hES cell research and abortion is also erroneous. Embryonic stem cells can be derived only for a very short period of time, during the blastocyst stage of embryo development, before the embryo has been implanted in the uterus. By the time the embryo starts to advance to the fetal stage of development in the womb, all of the cells from which embryonic stem cells can be derived have long ago differentiated into other cell types. In short, no embryonic stem cells exist in fetuses – these stem cells must be derived from the inner cell mass of a blastocyst before implantation and pregnancy have begun.

It should be admitted that the origins terminology gets much of its political power by being aligned simplistically and unjustifiably with the antiabortion movement. This conflation of hES cell research and abortion has been unfortunate, because it overlooks the possibility of an antiabortionist position that allows the use of stem cells derived from preimplantation fertility clinic embryos. According to many cultural and religious traditions, human embryos have no special moral status until they have been implanted in the womb and begun their development in conjunction with interactive biological cues from the maternal body.[5] Thus it would be no contradiction for some abortion opponents to support hES cell research, as long as – according to the dictates of their own values – these stem cells are obtained before pregnancy has begun. This more nuanced stance cannot be accommodated if one insists that the distinction between embryonic and adult stem cell research must be drawn along abortion lines.

But there are additional (perhaps more important) reasons for favoring the capabilities terminology of stem cells over the origins terminology, and I wish now to focus our attention on these matters. I propose that our analyses of the science and ethics of stem cell research will be deficient if we do not remain mindful of the fact that vital elements of human intervention lie at the heart of what makes stem cells so special. If we focus our attention on what stem cells are capable of doing rather than where they came from, we can better appreciate the insight that stem cells' capabilities are now coming to be defined more by scientists' manipulations in the laboratory than by the cells' innate biological

[5] According to Islamic and Jewish faith traditions, e.g., the embryo (or more specifically, the fetus) does not gain moral status until 40 days after implantation in the womb. The notion that moral status is conferred at conception is a relatively new idea in Roman Catholicism. St. Thomas Aquinas held that the fetus did not have a soul until the moment of quickening – i.e., when the motion of the fetus is perceived by the pregnant woman, usually 15 to 17 weeks after conception.

potentials. The origins terminology of *adult* and *embryonic* stem cells diverts our attention away from making this key observation.

Until just a few years ago there was no real practical distinction to be drawn between embryonic stem cells and pluripotent stem cells, for the only source of pluripotent stem cells at the time were from human and animal embryos created either through IVF or (in mice) through cloning – that is, somatic cell nuclear transfer (see Figure 2.4). Now, however, pluripotency can be engineered and directly introduced into nonpluripotent body cells in the laboratory. Due to recent advances in stem cell research, we now have *nonembryonic* pluripotent stem cells. These extraordinary advances (which I shall describe shortly) under-score just how artificial stem cells have become. Stem cells are not, to use a philosophical term of art, "natural kinds" as the origins terminology may imply. Rather, they become artificial tools for scientific discovery the moment they are plucked from their normal biological context within the human body and maintained *ex corporeally*.

To elaborate, let us return to the question posed at the beginning of this section: "What are stem cells?" As I have explained, the typical response has been to define stem cells by their ability to self-renew and differentiate into more specialized cells. But this simple definition glosses over two very important considerations: (1) the largely socially determined plasticity of stem cells and (2) the scientific and philosophi-cal implications of this plasticity. In answering the question "What are stem cells?" in a more philosophical manner, we find ourselves prob-ing a fascinating territory first introduced more than a century ago. To appreciate what stem cells are in a deeper sense, we must first recall the significance of the advent of human tissue culture. Stem cell science is but a dramatic new step in what has been an ongoing exploration of the near limitless possibilities of *in vitro* cell research. To grasp fully what stem cells are, then, we should take a moment to glance over our shoul-ders at the history of science.

Although human pluripotent stem cell research has existed for more than a decade, the basic enabling conditions for stem cell research were established well more than a century ago. In 1907, an American embry-ologist named Ross Harrison developed a method of keeping embry-onic frog nerve tissue alive in small glass containers for long periods (Landecker 2007).[6] Although the "hanging-drop" preparation that

---

[6] My thoughts in this chapter about the scientific and philosophical implications of tissue culture are indebted to Landecker's excellent book.

Harrison utilized had been used decades earlier to observe microorganisms such as bacilli under a microscope, Harrison improved the technique through aseptic conditions to enable the direct observation of growing nerve fibers in real time (Harrison 1907). A short while later, Alexis Carrel and Montrose Burrows modified Harrison's method into a general technique for the cultivation of all tissues, normal and abnormal, animal and human. One of the important changes that Carrel and Burrows introduced was the possibility of serial tissue cultivation, which was accomplished by using cells from the original culture to create new, secondary cultures. Thus one-time tissue preparations could be expanded to a potentially limitless series of cultures derived from one original source. Carrel and Burrows coined the now commonplace term *tissue culture* to describe their revolutionary techniques (Carrel and Burrows 1911).

It is nearly impossible to overstate the scientific and philosophical impact of the development of tissue cultivation. Scientifically, Carrel and Burrow's tissue culture method greatly facilitated the then-burgeoning field of *in vitro* research, which supplemented *in vivo* (in the body) experimentation and the histological examination of stained, dead tissue. Unlike the latter two methods, tissue culture made directly observable previously hidden biological processes and events, such as the growth of nerve fibers (they grow outward from a central neuron) and the origin of heartbeat (heart cells beat autonomously and are not stimulated by the nervous system) (Landecker 2007). Prior to tissue culture, the only way of studying hidden processes was to sequentially dissect laboratory animals or embryos, stain and examine the tissue slices histologically, and infer what was happening across these sequential slides. Histological examination was nonideal, because it could only provide snapshots of processes, not a visual reel of how living tissues actually behaved. Thus debates over the growth of nerve fibers and the origin of heartbeat, for example, could not be settled until tissue culture made these hidden processes directly observable in a dish in real time.

Second, in addition to making unobservable processes observable, tissue cultures allowed the serial cultivation of cells for research, thus eliminating the need to return to the cell donor source for further study. So the move from *in vivo* research to *in vitro* research was literal and figurative. Cells could be removed from the body and placed into culture where they took on a life of their own, independent of the body. Furthermore, living cells could be grown outside the body, returned back into the donor source, transferred to a different host, combined with other cells, or mixed with different species. From the advent of tissue culture to the present, living cells and tissues have become objects of study in their own right.

Philosophically, tissue cultures also had an enormous impact on the scientists who utilized them and their audiences. Like the lifeless physical matter of the mechanical universe, as conceptualized by the scientific founders of the modern worldview, living matter, too, could be arranged and rearranged according to secular man's instrumental aims. The corpuscular bodies of Descartes's mechanistic physics had found their biological analogue in cultured cells. Complex biological systems could be reduced to their more basic cellular units *in vitro*, observed, and then put back together. Thus, by the early twentieth century, scientists began to realize that all of the mysterious, hidden processes of biological life could, at least in principle, be studied in the laboratory after having been stripped bare of all their premodern explanatory garb. In short, the advent of tissue culture further fueled a modern drive toward scientific materialist explanations. It enabled the pursuit of biological research hypotheses framed wholly under a modern physicalist's worldview.

Furthermore, the notion of *plasticity* – a concept usually applied to nonliving matter – could now be extended to living cells and tissues. Tissue cultivation allowed cells and tissues to be grown, radically manipulated, and shared with other researchers for seemingly countless uses. Unlike the plasticity of lifeless objects, however, the plasticity of living matter relied from the beginning on constant human intervention. Although biologically independent from the body, tissues and cells in culture came to be wholly dependent on the laboratory technicians responsible for feeding them and changing their culture media. Because of their constant need to be maintained *in vitro*, tissue cultures could be said without too much exaggeration to grow in a new type of body – the socially organized body of the laboratory (Landecker 2007). Thus the plasticity of living matter must be understood not as a property "intrinsic" to the thing but rather as a property derived largely from human aims.

Flash forward to the present. Stem cell research would not have been possible without the technical and philosophical possibilities of biological plasticity introduced by tissue culture research in prior decades. Thus, to understand what stem cells are, we must take into account their social and historical context.

Understood in this context, then, stem cells are cells that have an extraordinarily high degree of plasticity. This plasticity is not a unitary property but a complex result of powerful forces. It is produced by the confluence of two vectors: the biological properties of stem cells and the ongoing manipulations of laboratory technicians. Both of these factors are crucial – the biological and the social. Under normal circumstances the pluripotency of embryonic cells (their capacity to differentiate into all cell types) is quickly lost following the embryo's implantation in the womb. But when cells from the embryo's inner cell mass are placed in a dish, an embryonic stem cell line may result that maintains pluripotency and the ability to self-renew – but only because scientists routinely add specific growth promoters and pathway inhibitors to expand the number of cells and to prevent them from differentiating into other cell types.[7]

According to the origins terminology, stem cells are naturally occurring entities that are known by their role in embryonic development and adult tissue repair. However, according to the capabilities terminology, what matters most about stem cells is their instrumental future, not their original biological function. Once stem cells are harvested and placed in a culture dish, they offer the benefits that typically accompany tissue culture systems. These benefits are numerous. Serial cultivation allows scientists to expand the number of stem cells *in vitro* from a single derivation and share them with researchers all around the world. Stem cells can be used to observe hidden developmental processes; and when they are derived from unhealthy donors, they can help researchers understand why diseased cells fail to grow and function properly. Thus stem cells *in vitro* allow scientists to bolster their understanding of human development as a cascade of physical events. Developmental biologists can use stem cells like living building blocks that can be mixed, matched, and transferred into hosts of the same or different species. Translational medical researchers can use stem cells as screening tools for drug development or as medical products that can be further shaped and ultimately delivered to patients.

To summarize, pluripotency should be viewed as the contemporary limit case of the plasticity of cells first introduced by the advent of tissue cultivation.[8] Once we admit that the full capabilities of stem cells in

---

[7] E.g., human pluripotent stem cells require FGF and activin/Nodal signaling to maintain their pluripotency *in vitro*. In contrast, cultures of mouse pluripotent stem cells require LIF signaling through the JAK/STAT3 signaling pathway (Paul Tesar, personal communication). Without pathway inhibitors or activators, pluripotent stem cells soon begin differentiating into specialized cells. Thus one might say that the default biological setting of stem cells is their tendency to lose their pluripotency.

[8] My emphasis here on pluripotent stem cells rather than multipotent stem cells is intentional. As I suggest in the next section the distinction between pluripotent and

culture depend on constant human intervention, it is not a far further step to accept the possibility that this plasticity could be engineered into fully differentiated cells. With the arrival of induced pluripotent stem (iPS) cell research, we find ourselves directly confronted with the realization that the full capabilities of stem cells are socially, not just biologically, determined.[9]

## Induced Pluripotent Stem Cells

Induced pluripotent stem cells are fully differentiated body cells (skin, peripheral blood cells, gut cells, etc.) that have been "reprogrammed" in the laboratory to take on the properties of embryonic stem cells (self-renewal and pluripotency). The idea of dedifferentiating somatic cells has existed for several decades (Gurdon et al. 1958; Wilmut et al. 1997). What was unexpected, however, was how easy this process would prove to be. The technique for creating iPS cells was pioneered in 2006 by Shinya Yamanaka and colleagues in Kyoto, Japan. The inspiration for this breakthrough came from a 2005 study from Harvard where researchers (using private funds) fused human body cells with hES cells (Cowan et al. 2005). Surprisingly, these fused cells began to act in their entirety like hES cells. The Japanese scientists reasoned that there must be something about hES cells that "teach" the body cells to act as they do.[10] So, rather than fusing cells together to get this result, Yamanaka's team used retroviruses to insert various combinations of stem cell–associated genes into mouse skin cells (fibroblasts) to see if pluripotency could be directly induced into these differentiated cells. Yamanaka and colleagues discovered that mouse fibroblasts could be reprogrammed to behave like mouse embryonic stem cells through the use of just four transcription

---

multipotent stem cells ceases to be very meaningful given the broader notion of plasticity I am advancing in this chapter and the advent of induced pluripotency, which renders any type of cell potentially pluripotent.

[9] Unlike traditional tissue cultures, however, where the cells were simply maintained and expanded, stem cells in culture are much more radically manipulated. These radical manipulations can create some skepticism over the degree to which the behavior of stem cells and their derivatives *in vitro* actually represent hidden biological processes and are not themselves artifacts of the manipulations. As the socially determined aspects of plasticity increase proportionately over the innate biological aspects, so too may the doubt that cells in culture provide an accurate window for observing hidden biological events in the body. This is a crucial point, which we will return to in the last few sections of this chapter.

[10] ShinyaYamanaka, personal communication.

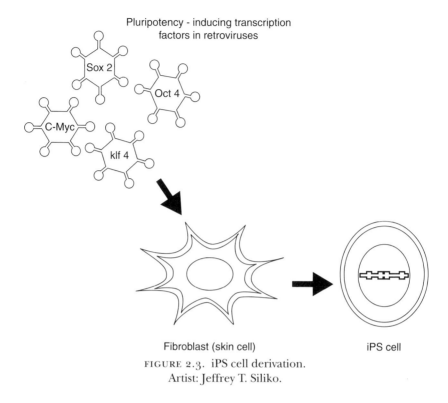

FIGURE 2.3. iPS cell derivation.
Artist: Jeffrey T. Siliko.

factors, now widely referred to as the "Yamanaka factors" – *Oct4*, *Sox2*, *Klf4*, and *c-Myc* (see Figure 2.3) (Takahashi and Yamanaka 2006).

*Oct4* and *Sox2* produce gene-regulatory proteins that help maintain the characteristics of embryonic stem cells. *Klf4* inhibits embryonic stem cell differentiation and cell death, and *c-Myc* (a gene associated with cancer) contributes to cell pluripotency and continued cell replication. When mouse iPS cells were made through this technique, they were able to self-renew and differentiate into cells representing each of the three germ lineages. And like embryonic stem cells, mouse iPS cells were able to form teratomas (masses of mixed differentiated tissues) when transplanted into immune-deficient mice, thus suggesting their induced pluripotency. Later, Yamanaka's team and others showed that mouse iPS cells could act like embryonic stem cells in terms of their ability to create adult chimeric mice and entire embryos using tetraploid complementation[11] (Maherali et al. 2007; Okita et al. 2007; Wernig et al. 2007; Zhao et al. 2009).

[11] The chimera assay is a rigorous standard for pluripotency. Mouse stem cells are removed from blastocyst A and tagged with a green florescent protein (GFP) marker. Then the

A short time after the mouse iPS cell breakthrough, teams led by Yamanaka, James Thomson, and George Daley each independently showed that human body cells could also be reprogrammed using a similar approach (Park et al. 2007; Takahashi et al. 2007; Yu et al. 2007). Today, there are many different methods for inducing pluripotency in human body cells (which I discuss in the next section), and human iPS cell research has become a booming subspecialty of stem cell science.

The iPS cell advancement underscores two of my chief claims. First, the widespread use of the term *cellular reprogramming* in the current iPS cell literature reinforces my point that stem cells in culture are malleable in ways previously thought to be reserved for nonliving matter.[12] Second, the iPS cell revolution, like all great scientific advances, not only increases the range of human will over nature, but it also disrupts our tidy categories. For example, while iPS cell technology is typically used to transform body cells, it can also in be applied to multipotent stem cells to make them pluripotent. Thus even the distinction between multipotent and pluripotent stem cells is becoming less secure due to scientists' ability to augment the former cell type's capabilities.

GFP tagged stem cells are injected into viable mouse blastocysts B, C, and D. Blastocysts B, C, and D are then implanted into a mouse uterus and allowed to come to term. If the A stem cells are pluripotent, then the resulting mouse pups should be chimeric – i.e., pup 1 should be composed of A and B cells; pup 2 should be composed of A and C cells; and pup 3 should be composed of A and D cells. The resulting mouse pups are acutely chimeric if they glow green from head to toe under a black light. Thus it can be concluded in this experiment whether the GFP-tagged A stem cells are pluripotent and can contribute to every organ and tissue system in the chimeric mice. An even better result is if the breeding of GFP-tagged chimeric mice results in the birth of other GFP-tagged mice, because this would show that the A stem cells were able to differentiate into functional sperm and eggs in the first generation and then were passed on to the second generation (germline transmission).

The tetraploid complementation assay is an even more stringent test for pluripotency. Two mammalian embryos are electrofused together at the two-cell stage so that both cells collapse into one another creating a single cell with a 4n genome (a cell with two sets of every chromosome). Candidate diploid pluripotent stem cells from another organism are then injected into the tetraploid blastocyst, which is then implanted in an experimental animal's uterus. If the transferred stem cells are truly pluripotent, then they will exclusively form a proper fetus, while the extraembryonic tissues, such as the placenta, will be exclusively formed by the tetraploid cells.

[12] Recently, scientists have been able to directly transdifferentiate specialized cells (such as skin cells) into other kinds of specialized cells without first transforming the starting cell into a pluripotent state. This is called direct transdifferentiation, and it has worked to create beta cells, neurons, heart cells, blood cells, and liver cells (Huang et al. 2011; Ieda et al. 2010; Pang et al. 2011; Szabo et al. 2010; Zhou et al. 2008). Neither these directly transdifferentiated cells nor their originators are stem cells. This is the latest and most extreme version of cellular reprogramming.

## Induced Pluripotent Stem Cells vs. Human Embryonic Stem Cells

Although stem cell scientists have roundly hailed iPS cell research as a major advance for the field as a whole, the arrival of iPS cells has caused much confusion among policy makers and the public regarding the need to continue scientific research using hES cells. Due to their (relatively) uncontroversial source, iPS cells have been touted by conservative opponents of hES cell research and the media as obviating the need for any further work on stem cells derived from human embryos (Associated Press 2007; Caulfield and Rachul 2011; Kass 2008).

This position is scientifically and ethically unwarranted. Despite rapid progress made with iPS cells, it is a serious mistake to jump to the conclusion that developments in iPS cell research make hES cell research unnecessary (Hyun et al. 2007).[13] Before I discuss the vast array of scientific uses of pluripotent stem cells in the following section, it is necessary that I explain here the reasons why (many of them quite technical) iPS and hES cell research must proceed together (Hyun et al. 2010).

There are many uncertainties surrounding iPS cells at this time. First, stem cell scientists today simply do not know whether human iPS cells have the exact same potential as hES cells. Human iPS cells resemble hES cells to a large extent in gene expression, epigenetic signature, and much functional pluripotency. Nevertheless, small differences in gene expression patterns have been observed between iPS and hES cells, and the exact nature of these differences is not yet well understood (Kiskinis and Eggan 2010). Second, although human iPS cells appear to be pluripotent in *in vivo* pluripotency assays (i.e., teratoma formation in mice), there is still a big question as to whether those cells, especially selected and examined by the current methods, can differentiate into all or certain specific fully functional cell types. Recent studies have suggested that iPS cells retain their epigenetic "memory" of their body cells of origin, thus making them possibly more resistant to differentiating into cell types of different germ lineages (Kim et al. 2010; Polo et al. 2010). Continued research is necessary with iPS and hES cells to better

---

[13] I wrote this commentary with Shinya Yamanaka, Rudolf Jaenisch, and Konrad Hochedlinger immediately after President Bush vetoed a congressional bill to expand federal funding for hES cell research. During the signing of his veto, Bush declared he felt justified in opposing the bill because of new research that showed that skin cells could be made into embryonic-like stem cells, thus bypassing the need for more hES cell research.

understand these differences and their implications for the development of iPS cell–derived applications.

Furthermore, very few published hES cell lines have been derived under conditions that may be appropriate for their eventual clinical application, and the technologies for stem cell maintenance and propagation are constantly improving (Hasegawa 2010). So while questions over the biological equivalence of iPS cell lines still need to be sorted out, scientists' efforts to optimize the development of pluripotent stem cells for clinical use will have to proceed using new populations of hES cells. For example, the first hES cell lines were established and cultured in media supplemented with 10 percent to 20 percent fetal calf serum on mouse embryonic fibroblast feeder layers (Thomson et al. 1998). Such widely used culture media introduce possible contamination by animal (xeno) agents. The use of human feeder layers, however, while avoiding xeno contamination, may introduce ambiguity in any subsequent genetic analysis of the hES cell line. Thus establishing xeno-free and feeder-free culture and expansion systems for hES cells continues to be a goal for the stem cell field.

One study has suggested, however, that feeder-free cultivation is associated with more stem cell chromosomal instability than conventional feeder systems (Catalina et al. 2008). If this is the case, then it would be important to discover exactly which culture conditions would improve the chromosomal stability of stem cells *in vitro*. This is no easy task, because little is known about genetic and epigenetic variation among different existing hES cell lines and how this variation affects the ability of hES cells to differentiate into particular cell types. So before one can determine what culture conditions best improve chromosomal stability, one must wrestle loose from the Catch-22 of having first to understand the average "natural" baseline of different hES cell lines' genetic stability – but by using cell lines that have unfortunately already been maintained in one culture system or another all along. Sorting through these conundrums will have to be done using hES cells and not iPS cells, because the latter have undergone a tremendous amount of genetic manipulation that may contribute to further genetic instability.

For the reasons stated earlier (and others that I discuss later), scientists do not believe it is safe to transplant the derivatives of iPS cells into humans at this time. Worse still, there are critical safety concerns about the techniques used to generate iPS cells. Specifically, the virus-mediated delivery of reprogramming factors is unacceptable for therapeutic purposes – because it could result in harmful genetic alterations and the permanent integration of cancer-causing agents called oncogenes (e.g., any of the four Yamanaka factors). Human embryonic stem cells, by contrast, have not been genetically manipulated and therefore offer a "purer" starting point for developing stem cell–based therapies. Thus continued hES cell research is vitally important to translate basic stem cell knowledge into clinically relevant interventions and perhaps later to pave the way for similar iPS cell–based therapies (Hyun et al. 2010).

It should be noted, however, that some key advances aimed at overcoming these safety concerns have been achieved recently by using non-integrating gene delivery approaches (such as adenovirus or episomal plasmid transfection), using cell-penetrating recombinant proteins and small molecules to induce the reprogramming, and using synthetic messenger RNA (Kim et al. 2009; Okita et al. 2008; Stadtfeld et al. 2008; Warren et al. 2010; Yu et al. 2009; Zhou et al. 2009). In any case, reprogramming body cells into iPS cells is slow under any of these conditions. These slow kinetics could present hidden risks in these lab-made cells, such as the accumulation of subtle genetic and epigenetic abnormalities during the reprogramming process, where cell growth pathways are activated and tumor suppressor pathways are overcome (Li et al. 2009). Furthermore, the current reprogramming process involved in the generation of iPS cells is still poorly understood and may entail fundamentally different mechanisms from other more robust reprogramming methods (e.g., somatic cell nuclear transfer), and consequently may harbor unknown safety concerns.

All of these scientific uncertainties necessitate the ongoing need for hES cell research. Crucially, the scientific reasons for continuing work in both iPS and hES cell research also serve to bolster the ethical reasons for advancing these two areas of stem cell science simultaneously. Not only must researchers use hES cells as controls for iPS cell studies, but also the safety concerns surrounding iPS cells require a far better understanding of the differences between these two stem cell types before proceeding to the clinic. One of the chief justifying reasons for conducting human stem cell research is to develop new therapeutic advances that may eventually help patients with intractable medical conditions. But before derivatives of iPS cells can be introduced into patients during the course of an early stage clinical trial, researchers and regulators alike must do their due diligence to ensure that the risks and effects of iPS cell technologies are well understood. This prerequisite understanding would be inadequate if hES cell research were to stop today (Hyun et al. 2010).

None of these points is intended to imply that hES cell research should be seen merely as a handmaiden to iPS cell research. Human embryonic stem cell research is an important endeavor in its own right. There remain invaluable and irreplaceable areas in hES cell research that cannot be conducted using iPS cells.

For example, hES cells are significantly different from mouse embryonic stem (ES) cells in terms of cell behaviors, gene expression, and signaling responses in self-renewal and differentiation, but correspond very closely to mouse epiblast stem cells (EpiSCs) that are derived from the postimplantation egg cylinder stage epiblasts of the mouse (Brons et al. 2007; Sato et al. 2003; Tesar et al. 2007). These observations support the notion that EpiSCs and hES cells are intrinsically similar and raise an attractive hypothesis that mouse ES cells and EpiSCs/hES cells represent two distinct cellular states: the mouse ES cell-like state representing the preimplantation inner cell mass and EpiSC-like state representing late epiblast cells, respectively. However, whether authentic mouse ES cell-like hES cells could be derived from human blastocysts remains to be explored (Najm et al. 2011). Derivation of the mouse ES cell-like hES cells would have significant value in both basic research and practical applications. These cells would be very useful to study early human development that may not be easily pursued otherwise. In addition, compared to mouse ES cells, EpiSCs and hES cells require more challenging *in vitro* culture conditions and differentiate poorly toward certain lineages. Mouse ES cell-like hES cells may represent a more robust pluripotent state with better self-renewal/survival and differentiation properties.

As this example highlights, advances in hES cell research continue to depend on advances in other scientific endeavors such as mouse stem cell research, just as iPS cell research has evolved in recent history from advances in our understanding of mouse ES and hES cells. As the advancement of stem cell science has shown time and time again, when science proceeds, it proceeds together as a group of interrelated activities. The politically motivated notion that one area of stem cell science can advance while ceasing (for nonscientific reasons) activity in another area is one that fails to makes much sense to the scientific mind. This crucial point is often lost in the political rhetoric surrounding iPS cell research. In an attempt to rebut such conservative political rhetoric, some proponents of hES cell research may appeal to a door metaphor when advocating continued activity in all areas of stem cell science: that is, one never knows behind which door the next big development may lie, so we ought to leave no door unopened. I believe perhaps a more

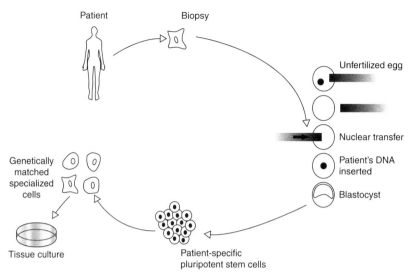

FIGURE 2.4. Somatic cell nuclear transfer.
Artist: Jeffrey T. Siliko.

accurate version of the metaphor is this: behind each door lies clues as
to which other doors to open next, thus facilitating the speed at which
researchers eventually unlock the next big development. The doors of
scientific inquiry are interconnected.

Consider one more example that helps illustrate this point. In addition
to iPS cell technology, pluripotent stem cells could also be obtained by the
process of somatic cell nuclear transfer (SCNT), a technique also referred
to as "research cloning" (*viz.*, by removing the DNA of an unfertilized egg
and replacing it with the DNA of a patient's body cell, researchers may be
able to produce embryonic stem cells that are genetically matched to the
patient and his or her particular disease – see Figure 2.4.)

Although it is technically challenging and raises ethical concerns for
many people, SCNT technology represents a different reprogramming
method and may produce pluripotent cells with different properties.[14]
Furthermore, investigations into SCNT mechanisms may also contribute to the development of better reprogramming methods by defined

---

[14] Recent attempts at human SCNT show that this process is scientifically extremely challenging (Noggle et al. 2011). Noggle and colleagues could not get their SCNT embryos
to divide normally to the blastocyst stage unless they left in the maternal nucleus in the
unfertilized eggs prior to SCNT. As a result, each of the resulting SCNT-derived stem
cells was triploid (i.e., had three copies of each genome – two from the somatic cell
donor and one from the egg donor).

factors. For example, the oocyte (unfertilized egg) reprograms the somatic cell nucleus within hours, whereas iPS cell reprogramming usually occurs over a period of weeks and may generate cells with accumulated harmful genetic and epigenetic changes (Barrilleaux and Knoepfler 2011). Somatic cell nuclear transfer could reveal faster, safer ways to reprogram somatic cells. Eggs are endowed with very high concentrations of unknown proteins involved in chromatin decondensation, DNA demethylation, and transcriptional activation of embryo genes (Jullien et al. 2011). Unveiling these proteins will help scientists improve the speed and safety of direct cellular reprogramming. This is important because troubling differences have recently been observed in gene expression patterns between iPS and hES cells (Barrilleaux and Knoepfler 2011). If, with continued SCNT research, normal SCNT stem cells can be derived, it would be extremely valuable to compare them to iPS cells and hES cells to understand key differences in each and their implications for the development of safer stem cell–based clinical applications.

Research cloning remains even more controversial than hES cell research, and I shall not delve here into the ethical reasons pro and con for SCNT (Hyun 2006b; Hyun and Jung 2006).[15] However, it should be recognized that the advancement of iPS cell research today should not affect the ethical permissibility of hES cell research. Undoubtedly, hES cell research remains controversial for a vocal minority,[16] and many opponents would argue that it should not continue if it can be replaced with less controversial means of advancing stem cell research and the clinical applications of stem cell science. Other critics would insist that hES cell research is permissible only if there is no other way to pursue a particular and important research question. But as I have pointed out in the preceding text, iPS cell research does not meet the necessary conditions for

Although these triploid SCNT pluripotent stem cells are not directly translatable for clinical applications, there are many valuable lessons we can learn from egg-mediated nuclear reprogramming (Daley 2011). As a case in point, Yamanaka and colleagues recently learned that the maternal transcription factor *Glis1* (which is enriched in unfertilized eggs and zygotes) could be used to replace the tumorigenetic transcription factor *c-Myc* to create iPS cells. Considering earlier cloning and chromosome transfer studies in the mouse (Egli et al. 2007; Wilmut et al. 1997) Yamanaka and colleagues reasoned that there may be transcription factors in unfertilized eggs and zygotes that promote nuclear reprogramming, and they identified *Glis1* as one of these key factors.

[15] I had written previously about the biological limitations of human SCNT and their implications for human reproductive cloning and the moral status of human SCNT embryos. See Hyun and Jung (2006).

[16] E.g., a recent poll shows that 72% of U.S. adults favor federal funding for hES cell research (Research!America 2010).

hES cell substitutability. Given this reality, iPS cell research should not be co-opted for political or ideological purposes. Although it is a truism that politics and public opinion often impact the direction of science in the real world, ideologically driven science policy should not be so misinformed as it appears to be in the case of proposing that iPS cell research continue at the expense of hES cell research. Such a policy would be detrimental to the stem cell field and could be dangerous for human research subjects and patients (as I discuss in later chapters). Human research subjects and patients should not be exposed to unnecessary risks attributable to the uncertainties surrounding iPS cells – uncertainties that must be answered through corresponding hES cell research. The reasons for continuing hES cell research are scientifically and ethically warranted.

In summary, recent progress in iPS cell research would not be possible without many years of research in hES cells. The iPS cell research field is still in its infancy. The international community of stem cell scientists has agreed that its further development is still highly dependent on the improved understanding of hES cells (International Society for Stem Cell Research 2008b). The caravan of stem cell science is composed of many parts, yet it must proceed together as a whole.

## The Role of Stem Cells in Biomedical Research

Throughout this chapter I have suggested that pluripotent stem cells in culture are powerful research tools with varying degrees of artificiality. These manipulated cells play an extremely important role in basic and translational research. I continue in this section with a discussion of some major uses of pluripotent stem cells. Then I discuss examples of multipotent stem cell research and their relationships to pluripotent stem cells.

Pluripotent stem cells are used for scientific and biomedical research aims unattainable with multipotent stem cells. In basic research, they are used to help us understand healthy and unhealthy human development. For example, pluripotent stem cells are utilized to address fundamental questions in developmental biology, such as how primitive cells differentiate into each of the three germ layers and how different organ systems first come into being. By increasing our knowledge of human development, pluripotent stem cells may help us better understand important, fundamental problems, such as the causes of fetal deformations.

Straddling the middle of the continuum between basic and translational research is the use of pluripotent stem cells for disease modeling. By deriving and studying pluripotent stem cells that are genetically matched to diseases such as Parkinson's disease, researchers hope to map out the developmental course of complex medical conditions to understand how, when, and why diseased specialized cells fail to function properly in patients. A useful metaphor is this:[17] when a patient with a delayed, degenerative disease like Parkinson's is diagnosed in a clinic, she is like a jetliner that has already crashed to the ground. That is, by the time the symptoms of Parkinson's become apparent to the patient and the clinician, the disease has already progressed to a significantly advanced stage. Extracting and examining the patient's damaged neural cells at this point will not tell clinical investigators how or why her dopaminergic cells have failed to function properly. Attempting to learn about the disease process in this manner would be analogous to arriving at a crash site and piecing together the fuselage to try to figure out why it crashed. This would not be a very informative endeavor. What one needs to recover instead is the flight data recorder to understand precisely how, when, and why the plane hurtled to earth. Analogously, disease-specific stem cells offer researchers a "flight data recorder" for degenerative diseases. By modeling and studying the developmental course of complex diseases in a dish, researchers may be able to observe cell-intrinsic defects that would improve our understanding of why and how certain diseases entail the loss of cell function (see Figure 2.5) (Daley 2010).

In the way that tissue cultivation in the early 1900s allowed scientists to move hidden biological processes into a culture dish, the derivation of disease-specific pluripotent stem cells today allows researchers to move a degenerative disease from the patient and into a dish for direct observation. Disease-in-a-dish modeling systems thus provide researchers with a method for studying human diseases previously unavailable through animal research alone or histological examination of dead, stained tissue.

Stem cell scientists have succeeded in producing a few disease-specific stem cell lines using unwanted fertility clinic embryos that had been tested positive for serious genetic diseases, such as cystic fibrosis and spinal muscular atrophy. However, no embryo genetic screening methods exist for complex diseases such as Parkinson's disease and Alzheimer's; thus scientists must develop their own disease-specific stem cell lines for these and many other diseases they wish to study.

---

[17] I owe this jetliner metaphor to Lawrence Goldstein.

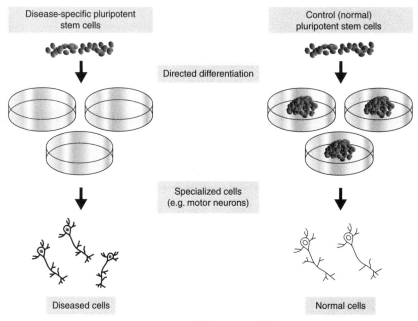

FIGURE 2.5.  Disease modeling.
Artist: Jeffrey T. Siliko.

Now iPS cells have arrived on the scene. Since iPS cell research first began, it has attracted enormous interest with respect to its potential applications in biomedical research. That is, by utilizing reprogramming techniques using body cells from donors with specific diseases, disease-tailored pluripotent stem cells could be obtained and further differentiated into functional cells for drug screens or cell-based therapies with alleviated immunocompatibility issues.[18] The ease at which disease- and patient-specific pluripotent stem cells can now be generated signifies an enormous advance for stem cell science. Human iPS cell technology allows researchers to study patients' diseases by comparing the developmental course of patients' iPS cells with iPS cells derived from healthy volunteers. For diseases that have a particular cellular phenotype, such as

---

[18] It must be noted, however, that two considerations challenge the hope of one day using patient-specific iPS cells on the patients from which they were derived. The first concerns FDA issues, which I discuss later in this chapter (see note 22). The second concerns a recent published study that showed an auto-immune reaction in mice when they had their own iPS cells transferred back into them (Zhao 2011). This finding casts some doubt on the notion that derivatives of patients' iPS cells could be autologously transferred without rejection.

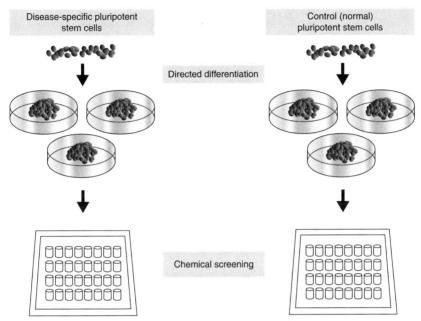

FIGURE 2.6. Drug screening and development.
Artist: Jeffrey T. Siliko.

sickle cell anemia and immunodeficiency, iPS cells derived from patients can be differentiated in a dish to reveal developmental pathologies when compared to the development of normal cells differentiated from healthy iPS cell populations. Just a short time after the advent of human iPS cells, researchers were able to derive disease-specific iPS cell lines for just this purpose from patients suffering from Lou Gehrig's disease, as well as from patients suffering from many other conditions, such as juvenile type 1 diabetes and Parkinson's disease (Dimos et al. 2008; Park et al. 2008).

Furthermore, iPS cell-derived disease model systems could enable pharmaceutical researchers to quickly screen chemical libraries to identify drugs that might restore normal cell activity in diseased cells (see Figure 2.6).

Researchers can aggressively test the safety and efficacy of new targeted drug interventions on tissue cultures of living human cells derived from disease-specific pluripotent stem cells, thus reducing the risks associated with human subjects research and lowering development costs. It is estimated that less than 11 percent of all experimental drugs make it through the clinical trials process to the marketplace, at a cost of U.S. $1.2 to 1.7 billion per drug (Kaitin 2008; Sollano et al. 2008). In 2001, clinical trials were halted with 30 percent of experimental drugs because of lack of efficacy and in another 30 percent due to high toxicity, usually to the heart and/or liver (Laustriat 2010). Healthy iPS cells could in principle be differentiated into cardiomyocytes (heart cells) and hepatocytes (liver cells) to help analyze *in vitro* the probable toxic side effects of drugs.

However, to leverage iPS cell technology into either of these pharmaceutical applications – targeted drug development and toxicity screening – stem cell scientists must first tackle at least three challenges (Inoue and Yamanaka 2011).

First, researchers must improve their technical ability to directly and reliably differentiate iPS cells into high numbers of specialized cells of interest, while minimizing iPS cells' propensity for tumorigenicity (tendency to form tumors). All of these are challenges facing the use of any pluripotent stem cells. Whether one is using iPS cells or hES cells, pluripotent stem cells need to do exactly what researchers want them to do and not spin out of control and form unwanted cell types.

An often-overlooked element of stem cell differentiation is the complex role that a stem cell's microenvironment (or niche) plays. Exactly how the stem cell niche environment influences stem cell differentiation is incompletely understood, but all attempts to reliably and safely direct pluripotent stem cells to differentiate into wanted specialized cells must ultimately recapitulate the complex and dynamic signals of the stem cell niche environment (Peerani and Zandstra 2010). Stem cell–niche engineering *in vitro* must be accomplished by calling upon bioengineers to create local microenvironments for stem cells in a reliable, controlled, and reproducible manner. Some of these *in vitro* microenvironments may have to be three-dimensional, with complex mechanical features and scaffolds. For example, research into embryonic heart development has suggested that shear forces from blood flow may be necessary for the proper development of the hematopoietic (blood) system (Adamo et al. 2009; North et al. 2009).

Second, for diseases that have an onset during a later stage of life, such as neurodegenerative diseases like Lou Gehrig's disease and Parkinson's, disease-specific iPS cell-derived body cells (neural cells, e.g.) may not immediately manifest the disease phenotype without the presence of environmental cues and stressors, which, like the cells' niche environment, must somehow also be replicated *in vitro*.

Third, a challenge is that the notions of a control population of "healthy" iPS cells need further thought and refinement. Genomewide association studies have recently shown that every individual has disease-relevant single-nucleotide polymorphisms (Satake et al. 2009). Thus it would be impossible to categorically identify any iPS cells that are a perfect nondisease control (Inoue and Yamanaka 2011). Faced with this reality, iPS cell researchers will have to propose a definition of "control" iPS cells either deductively (e.g., using diseased iPS cells with and without a disease-correcting genetic modification) or inductively (e.g., using iPS cells from a patient with disease X and a disease X–free family member) (Inoue and Yamanaka 2011).

Assuming these three challenges can be adequately met, pluripotent stem cells can have a powerful role in developmental biological research, disease modeling, and drug development. Furthermore, stem cells have a wide range of other possible uses for translating basic knowledge into clinical applications. For many types of diseases and injuries, the path from bench to bedside is paved by a dynamic interaction between pluripotent and multipotent stem cell research. Both stem cell types are crucial for the road to clinical translation. Take, for instance, just four areas of clinically relevant stem cell research: skeletal muscle repair, cardiovascular disease, neurodegenerative disease, and cancer stem cells.

Skeletal muscle has the ability to regenerate new muscle fibers after injury. Alexander Mauro discovered in 1961 that the most important cells for skeletal muscle regeneration are a type of myogenic progenitor cell located between the basal lamina and the plasma membrane around each muscle fiber (Mauro 1961). Mauro called these progenitor cells satellite cells. Today these cells are believed to be key to understanding the mechanisms for skeletal muscle regeneration (Tedesco 2010). The expansion and study of satellite cells *in vitro* may help researchers develop cell therapies for diseases caused by skeletal muscle degeneration, such as muscular dystrophy. Unfortunately, satellite cells are difficult to isolate and maintain in culture (where they appear to lose their "stemness"). If pluripotent stem cells could be differentiated directly into satellite cells, then there could be an abundant supply of regenerative cells that could be used to discover how to use them for muscle repair. Learning how to create myogenic progenitor cells, such as satellite cells, from stem cells will require a combined knowledge of pluripotent and multipotent cell types.[19]

---

[19] A very important concept here is "clinical scale" – i.e., whether one is able to obtain enough cells to provide a therapy (Willy Lensch, personal communication). Burn victims usually have preserved skin on the underside of their arms and in their groin area. However, it may often be insufficient in mass or area to cover the burned regions.

Unlike skeletal muscle, the heart is greatly limited in its ability to heal itself. The creation of new functional cardiomyocytes (cardiac cells that are destroyed by myocardial infarction) is a primary goal for cardiovascular medicine (Yi 2010). Cardiomyocytes could be made either from differentiated pluripotent stem cells or by stimulating the limited inherent regenerative capacity of the heart. The first approach would use pluripotent stem cells to create transplantable cardiomyocytes. The latter would use pluripotent stem cell derivatives as catalysts to trigger the heart's multipotent cardiac stem cells to make their own cardiomyocytes. For example, a recent study has shown proof-of-principle in the mouse model that the adult heart has a resident stem or progenitor cell population that can create fully differentiated cardiomyocytes. Now the goal is to discover ways to activate these cell populations to target and heal damaged areas of the heart (Smart et al. 2011). Either of these approaches will require expanded stem cell knowledge of the fundamental biology of heart progenitor cells, their microenvironmental niche, and the mechanisms for progenitor cell homing and migration to injured sites.

Spinal cord injury and neurodegenerative diseases, such as Parkinson's disease, Alzheimer's disease, and Lou Gehrig's disease are devastating for patients who have little or no recourse from their conditions. Stem cell–based approaches could involve the replacement of lost or damaged neurons and glial cells by the direct transplantation of stem cell derivatives developed *in vitro* or by the inducement of exogenous multipotent stem cells in the CNS to release neuroprotective responses (Lindvall and Kokaia 2010). Besides facilitating our understanding of the pathogenesis of neurodegenerative disorders and the development of new drugs through disease-in-a-dish model systems, pluripotent stem cell derivatives may one day be used for neurotransplantation therapies. For example, primary neural tissue from aborted fetuses has been used for transplantation in patients with Parkinson's disease and Huntington's disease with some positive results (Lindvall et al. 2004; Lindvall and Kokaia 2010).[20] However, many of the grafts did not survive and few

---

The same goes for umbilical cord blood that contains enough hematopoietic stem cells to transplant a child. If the numbers or scale of these cells could be amplified, an existing therapy could be offered with a much-greater chance for success. Clinical scale comes into the pluripotent stem cell arena as one can grow enormous amounts of them on the front end and then differentiate them forward to cell types that are difficult or impossible to amplify in number, such as cardiomyocytes.

[20] There has been considerable debate regarding the results of these studies. I discuss this controversy in Chapter 7.

patients had established reasonable functional recovery. Researchers believe that one of the main reasons for these inconsistent results may be the heterogeneity of the donor tissue. In these early studies, neural cells from several fetuses were pooled for each transplant recipient (Koch et al. 2009). To increase the number of neural cells available for transplant and to standardize their quality, researchers need an expandable source of neural tissue. Pluripotent stem cell–derived cells, such as dopaminergic neurons for Parkinson's disease patients, may provide this much-needed source. To pursue this strategy, pluripotent stem cell–derived neural cells will have to be functionally compared to neural cells obtained post mortem.

Another major area in which stem cell research may have an important clinical impact is in the study of cancer stem cells. Cancer stem cells are a subpopulation of tumor cells that possess the capacity to self-renew and to generate heterogeneous lineages of cancer cells that make up the tumor (Frank et al. 2010). Conventional anticancer approaches have been directed mainly at bulk tumor populations. Some researchers believe that conventional cancer treatments are suboptimal because they do not target and destroy cancer stem cells, which go on to perpetrate tumorigenesis. Cancer stem cells must be destroyed or else tumors can reoccur. Targeting cancer stem cells could involve one of several different strategies, such as developing antitumor drugs that interfere with cancer stem cell pathways, or that target prospective markers of cancer stem cells, or that disrupt tumor-causing interactions in the cancer stem cell microenvironment (Frank et al. 2010). Each of these strategies will require increased knowledge of cancer stem cells and how they behave. If successful, cancer stem cell research could lead to new cancer therapies for malignancies that are refractory or currently resistant to conventional anticancer agents.

As these four examples suggest, the road to clinical translation from basic stem cell research to the clinic is promising and exciting. However, several very important and difficult scientific issues remain to be addressed. In the next section I elaborate further on the technical problems that lie ahead and the ethical questions that arise from them.

## Uncharted Territories

As I suggested earlier, stem cell–based clinical interventions can take one of several forms. More precisely, these interventions can involve either (1) direct cell replacement using multipotent stem cells or new cells derived from pluripotent stem cells *in vitro*, or (2) indirect healing support through secretion of growth factors to stimulate local endogenous repair, homing signals that recruit the patient's own multipotent stem cells for repair, or homing signals that modulate the patient's immune system (Magnus et al. 2008).

Furthermore, depending on whether therapeutic cells are heavily manipulated before delivery to the patient, one of three models of cell therapy distribution will pertain (Ahrlund-Richter et al. 2009). It is fairly common for multipotent stem cells, such as blood stem cells, to be harvested from and returned to the same patient (autologous transfer) after minimal manipulation (defined as cells cultured under nonproliferating conditions for less than forty-eight hours). This "point of contact" distribution model is not subject to U.S. Food and Drug Administration (FDA) regulations. Autologous transfer of a patient's own minimally manipulated multipotent stem cells is considered a bedside service by the FDA and subject only to the professional norms of medical practice. For more-than-minimally manipulated cells, however (e.g., any pluripotent stem cells and their derivatives), these more complex biologic products are regulated by external agencies – for instance, in the United States by the FDA, in the European Union by the Advanced Therapies Regulation, and in the United Kingdom by the Human Tissue Authority (HTA).[21] In this case, one of two distribution models will apply: a cell banking model or a manufacturing model. For the remainder of this chapter I will focus on the banking and manufacturing models, and I will save for further discussion in Chapter 8 the point-of-contact clinical service model.[22]

---

[21] The FDA regulates any human cells or tissues that are "highly processed, are used for other than their normal function, are combined with non-tissue components, or are used for metabolic purposes" (Halme and Kessler 2006, 1730). The European Union's Advanced Therapies Regulation defines a *biological medicinal product* as product that "contains or consists of cells or tissues that have been subject to substantial manipulation so that biological characteristics, physiological functions or structural properties relevant for the intended clinical use have been altered, or of cells or tissues that are not intended to be used for the same essential function(s) in the recipient and the donor" (Part IV of Annex I to Directive 2001/83/EC).

[22] It should be noted that, despite claims to the contrary by the media and some stem cell researchers, the use of patient-specific iPS cells and their derivatives does *not* fall under the clinical service model. When iPS cells first arrived on the scene, many commentators enthused that these cells opened up the possibility of treating patients directly with their own reprogrammed cells without the threat of auto-immune rejection. This idealized picture of "personalized medicine" is seriously flawed for at least four reasons. First, due to their extreme manipulations in culture, iPS cells are considered complex biologic

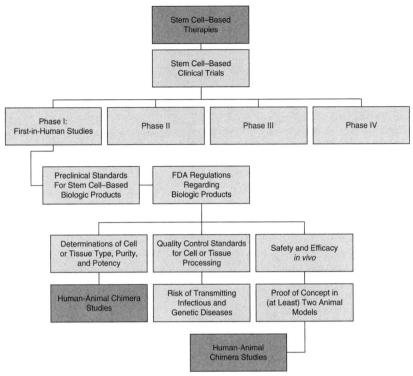

FIGURE 2.7. Food and Drug Administration flowchart.

Aside from the hematopoietic (blood) system and epithelial cells for skin replacement therapies, stem cells and their derivatives are novel biologic products for which scientists, clinicians, and regulators have very little experience in humans. Although the FDA has general preclinical requirements for complex biologic products (see Figure 2.7), it remains unclear at this time exactly how stem cell–based biologic products are to be prepared for their delivery into research subjects and patients.

products and must be regulated as such, thus obviating the possibility of point-of-contact delivery at the bedside. Second, because iPS cells are genetically modified they are doubly burdened by FDA regulatory approval requirements for gene therapy. Third, because each patient-specific iPS cell line is genetically distinct, each would be considered a separate investigational product requiring separate FDA approval. And finally, as mentioned earlier in this chapter (see note 18), a study showed that mouse iPS cells provoked an immune reaction when transferred back into the same genetic strain of mice from which they were derived, thus casting a cloud on the assumption that derivatives of patients' own iPS cells could be autologously transferred back into them without rejection.

Unlike pills, which are stable, uniform, and easily reproducible in mass quantities, stem cells and their derivatives are dynamic, living, biological entities that are difficult to scale up to huge numbers of specialized cells of uniform quality. Cells in culture tend to age and accumulate genetic and epigenetic changes, as well as changes in cell behavior. Unfortunately, scientists' understanding of the genetic stability of cells in culture is not well developed at this time, and tests for determining this stability are still evolving (Ahrlund-Richter et al. 2009).

Most pharmaceuticals are developed by companies with extensive experience manufacturing small molecule drugs and are overseen by an FDA (or FDA-like) process developed around drug marketing approval. In contrast, most stem cell–based products are initiated by researchers in academic laboratories or small biotechnical companies who may have very limited experience in developing manufacturing processes or in sourcing biological materials for cell therapies. This inexperience – coupled with a current lack of clear, stem cell–specific regulatory standards for highly manipulated stem cell products – raises complex ethical questions concerning informed consent by original donors, their autonomy rights, and the level of risk exposure for research subjects and patients. In order to develop stem cell–based therapies, we must enter uncharted territories. The following are just a few of these unfamiliar areas.

### Sourcing

Pills are manufactured from beginning to end. Living cells, by contrast, must first be sourced from donors. Sourcing cells requires the informed consent of tissue donors. The requirement for informed consent by tissue donors is not new, but what is novel for stem cell research is the potential need for long-term health monitoring of original donors. In addition to the usual donor screening procedures for infectious and genetic diseases, the development of stem cell–based therapies may require recontacting donors to gather additional health information down the road that may impact the quality and safety of their derived stem cell lines. For example, if cells or embryos are donated by persons who later are found to suffer from a genetic disorder, the resulting pluripotent stem cell lines may be unsuitable for differentiation into specialized cells for therapy (Halme and Kessler 2006). The traceability of a stem cell–based product to the original biological materials donor is important for safety reasons, but it also raises the need for counterbalancing confidentiality requirements to ensure donor privacy. Some jurisdictions already require traceability of stem cell products to their starting materials, so it is imperative now that stem cell researchers everywhere put into practice appropriate informed consent procedures to account for this requirement when sourcing cells.[23]

Furthermore, because stem cells must be derived from cells and tissues sourced from donors, ethical questions loom large regarding donors' ownership rights and other autonomy interests over stem cell lines and their derivatives. Historically, U.S. courts have favored guidelines for blood and organ donation and cell-line creation from tumor samples that grant all commercial rights to the investigator or hospital obtaining the biological materials with informed consent. The case of *Moore v. Regents of California* and litigation over the HeLa cell line are perhaps the most widely known examples of this legal viewpoint (Skloot 2010).[24] Although this may be the current legal standard in the United States, some may question whether this legal standard is ethically justified. Unlike other biological samples, pluripotent stem cells can be differentiated into all cell types for a variety of unforeseen future research uses that may be discomforting to donors; therefore, sourcing cells will require considerable planning and discussion with prospective donors to protect their autonomy and privacy rights.

The next set of issues pertains to the complexity and risk of transferring stem cell–based products into research subjects and patients. Before highly manipulated cells from one donor can either be banked or placed directly into another recipient (allogeneic transfer), the type of cell(s) being banked or transferred must first be well characterized. Exactly what kind of cells are in the therapeutic product? What is their purity and potency? Lack of clarity on these points can expose recipients to unknown and potentially grave risks.

## Determining Cell Type

Attempts to determine cell type can be scientifically contentious. Consider the classification of pluripotency. There are different tests available

---

[23] In the European Union, e.g., the traceability of biological medicinal products, including human cells or tissues, must be maintained for a minimum of 30 years after the expiry data of the product, or longer if deemed necessary (Regulation [EC] No. 726/2004, 13th November 2007, Article 15).

[24] HeLa was the first widely used human cell line. It was created from a cervical biopsy procured by Johns Hopkins Hospital from an African American cancer patient named Henrietta Lacks in 1951. The HeLa cell line was produced without her knowledge and was used for countless research and commercial uses, including the development of the polio vaccine. Neither Henrietta Lacks nor her family received royalties from the commercial success of the HeLa cell line.

to determine whether a population of stem cells is pluripotent.[25] A common standard is to see if candidate pluripotent stem cells can be differentiated *in vitro* into cells representing all three germ lineages. This is a reasonable test, but it is a bit like trying to determine the potential of a car by revving its engine in a garage. What one needs to know is how the thing behaves in a more dynamic environment. Thus a more rigorous standard for human stem cells is to see whether candidate pluripotent stem cells can form a teratoma (a lump of human tissues representing all three germ layers) when placed in the kidney capsule or other enclosed region of an immune-deficient mouse. Teratoma formation after two or three months suggests that the human stem cells are high quality and capable of expressing their pluripotent characteristics *in vivo*. The most that stem cell researchers can hope for at this point is that their human pluripotent stem cells pass the teratoma assay.

The take-home point from this discussion is that not all stem cells collected from human blastocysts or derived through the iPS cell process pass the teratoma assay, leading some in the stem cell community to conclude that some purported hES and iPS cell lines in existence today are not truly pluripotent.[26] The debate over which pluripotency assays should constitute the minimum requirements for the stem cell field is especially important in light of the fact that there are now several different approaches to inducing pluripotency in body cells and not all of them may result in stem cells that are capable of passing the teratoma assay. Depending on which assay one believes is absolutely required, some iPS cell lines (and some hES cell lines) may not be found to deserve the mantle of pluripotency, thus complicating the standards for accepting stem cell lines into master cell banks and repositories.

When it comes to specialized cells derived from hES or iPS cells, determining cell type can get even murkier. Cells manufactured through differentiation protocols or harvested and processed from different anatomical sites or from unrelated individuals present significant potential for biological variability. However, there are no widely agreed upon

---

[25] I discuss here just two of the four possible pluripotency assays (*in vitro* differentiation and the teratoma test), because these are the only ones currently used to test the pluripotency of human stem cells. The other two assays – the creation of chimeric offspring and tetraploid complementation – are only used to test mouse and other animal stem cells, because they involve the live birth of experimental offspring. See note 11.

[26] A few years ago, researchers in Italy claimed that they procured human pluripotent stem cells from amniotic fluid and the placenta (De Coppi et al. 2007); however, these cells did not pass the teratoma test, and most stem cell scientists do not wish to call these cells pluripotent (Lensch et al. 2007).

standards for what surrogate markers ought to be used to validate cell identity (Ahrlund-Richter 2009). This is unfortunate, because it is important to know exactly what type of individual cells and their relative proportions are present in a specific stem cell–based product. The ability to consistently and reliably identify cells within a specific stem cell–based product and across different products is an essential step for determining purity and safety. If there are undifferentiated stem cells or uncharacterized cells in the final product, then the risk of tumor and other unwanted tissue formation may be unacceptably high. During the development of small molecule drugs, it is possible to completely assess the active ingredient and purity of the product to a very high degree of accuracy. Even if major manufacturing changes are made, a drug product can still be shown to be comparable to a product manufactured through a previous process. In the case of stem cell–based products, analogous standards have yet to be agreed upon among researchers and centralized stem cell repositories.

*Purity and Potency*

It would be unrealistic to demand that a stem cell–based product be 100 percent pure – that is, for it to be comprised of all one desired, active cell type.[27] Not even pharmaceutical drugs can claim to be 100 percent pure. So the key question is how pure is "pure enough"? This is not simply an academic point. Cultures of neural stem cells, for example, are often contaminated with glial cells; and directly differentiated populations of hES cells can contain undifferentiated cells that could produce unintended effects – like malignancies – when transplanted. However, it may be desirable to have mixed populations of cell types in the final product to promote the best overall healing effect (as may be the case with bone marrow transplantation).

In light of these considerations, perhaps "contamination" is the more useful concept to employ here rather than "purity." Contaminants can include residual stem cells, cells that have differentiated into undesired cell types during processing, and feeder layer cells (Halme and Kessler 2006). Thus it is incredibly important for stem cell researchers to be able to identify and detect all cell types in a particular stem cell–based product, and, as I have acknowledged previously, researchers are not yet able

---

[27] In the case of bone marrow transplantation for leukemia, the donated graft is usually comprised of many different types of cells, many or most of which are not hematopoietic stem cells.

to determine all cell types, particularly ambiguous cell types that may have been produced during the manufacturing process for which there are no clear biological analogues for comparison.[28]

It should be acknowledged that considerations of cell product purity ought to include more than just the worry that a stem cell–based product may contain unwanted, contaminating cells. Unwanted changes to a cell product can also result from intrinsic changes to the cells over time. Cells in culture are in a constant state of flux. Changes can include changes in their mitochondria, methylation profiles, and other epigenetic and genetic alterations (Maitra et al. 2005). Many of these changes may be of little consequence, but others might lead to the activation of cancer genes (Ahrlund-Richter et al. 2009). An important task for manufacturers, cell bankers, and regulators is to define what types of changes within a (reasonably pure) population of cells is acceptable or "normal" given conditions for culturing and maintaining tissues.

Once a benchmark for acceptable change in culture has been defined, it is also imperative to set standards for expanding the number of wanted cells (scaling up) and shipping and freezing cells for delivery to the clinic. These latter issues, particularly shipping and freezing, tend to be ignored in discussions about the purity of stem cell–based products. It may prove difficult to maintain the quality of a stem cell–based product during its transfer to the end user. For example, motor neurons may need to be shipped live within a certain time frame from the manufacturing facility or cell bank (Ahrlund-Richter et al. 2009). Stem cell–based products may have to be packaged and maintained in very specific environmental conditions to ensure that the samples arrive healthy without additional accumulated changes. Historically, it took the blood bank industry and the organ transplantation community many years to develop their own optimal shipping practices. It could take stem cell product developers and central repositories at least the same amount of time, or even longer, to do the same.

Finally, stem cell–based biologic products have to have a known potency. Like the potency of a drug, the "potency" of a cell could be defined as some quantitative measure of that cell's desired biological activity or effect. How to measure cell potency, however, is an open question. Stem cells and their derivatives are dynamic, living entities whose behavior

---

[28] To make matters even more complex, even if all surrogate markers of cell identification could be agreed upon, the failure to detect a particular unwanted cell type does not prove that none of these unwanted cells are in the stem cell–based product.

in the body can be influenced by their particular niche microenvironments. Thus, although *in vitro* demonstration of cell activity may provide some evidence of potency, it may be necessary to assess the potency of a stem cell–based product in animal models, because cells may undergo major functional changes after transplantation. But what animal models are best for determining cell potency? How similar do the animals have to be to humans? These and other challenging ethical questions about animal research, including the use of nonhuman primates, will be the subject of Chapters 5 and 6.

In order to minimize the risks and uncertainties I have discussed in this section, the manufacture of stem cell–based products and the banking of master stem cell lines must be done under (yet to be universally agreed upon) good manufacturing practice (GMP), which is a form of quality assurance that aims to ensure that a product is consistently stored or produced, beginning with the starting materials, premises and equipment, and the training and hygiene of the staff. The GMP for stem cell–based biologic products will require widespread agreement within the international stem cell community as to what these standard practices ought to be, including the very early phases of hES or iPS cell derivation and cultivation. In the case of stem cell–based products, the nature of the therapeutic product can be highly dependent on derivation, culture, manufacture, storing, and shipping processes. Changes to any one of these practices could affect changes in important characteristics including how the product will behave in humans. For this reason, it is crucial that none of these "technical" details be shrugged off as unimportant for ethics, for they could have a huge impact on the safety of stem cell–based therapies. To reason intelligently about the ethics for stem cell research and its application in humans, one must be aware of the scientific issues surveyed in this chapter.

## Conclusion

I have argued that cultured stem cells are scientific tools with varying degrees of artificiality. Stem cells comprise an important strategic division in the modern physicalist's arsenal to survey and battle humankind's natural infirmities. Scientists can leverage stem cells to pursue questions in developmental biology, study and model human diseases, and develop and screen new pharmaceuticals. Stem cells can also be directly engineered and manipulated into complex stem cell–based products for new patient therapies. As research tools, stem cells are unlike conventional

tissue cultures of the past, which were not nearly as malleable. As therapeutic agents, stem cells occupy an uncertain place somewhere between
conventional drugs and transplantation. Contrary to what many people
may believe, the development of stem cell therapies does not track neatly
alongside the development of drugs. Nor are most proposed stem cell–
based therapies analogous to organ or tissue transplantation in any
straightforward sense, due to the former's additional differentiation and
proliferation in recipients. There is still so much to discover about how
stem cells can be used. Whether stem cells are used to advance the basic
biological sciences or are manufactured into clinically relevant products,
the caravan of stem cell research must proceed together as a whole.

The chief connecting link between each component of this caravan is
the combined biological and socially based plasticity of stem cells. It is
this remarkable and multifarious plasticity that makes stem cell research
so unique – a plasticity first introduced into living matter by Harrison,
Carrel, and Burrows, and later radically augmented by Yamanaka and his
contemporary iPS and hES cell researchers. This ever-increasing ability
to make living cells bend to our will is a newfound power that raises the
complementary possibilities of opportunity and danger. Regardless of
the new developments and techniques that are bound to emerge over
the next several years in stem cell research, this central defining characteristic of stem cells – their multifarious plasticity – will remain a constant
presence, as will the technical and ethical challenges that arise from it.

Science, as it has done since the seventeenth century, impels challenging ethical questions about what we ought to do in light of new uncertainties. The bioethics of stem cell research revolves largely around two foci:
(1) deontological considerations, such as the rights of original donors,
and the voluntary consent of research subjects and patients receiving
stem cell–based interventions; and (2) consequentialist considerations,
such as the broader social impacts of animal modeling and other preclinical methods to develop new stem cell–based therapies, and the risks associated with using highly manipulated, highly processed cells in humans.
Within this elliptical bioethical universe reverberates the echoes of many
old themes in research ethics. However, these old notes now beat across
an unfamiliar and rapidly shifting terrain of new scientific realities. Can
our time-tested principles and procedures of research ethics fulfill the
task of granting us appropriate control over the direction and speed of
stem cell science? This is the subject of the next two chapters.

# 3

## The Golden Bridle I

### *Philosophical Research Ethics*

According to Greek mythology, Athena, the goddess of wisdom, bestowed upon the mortal Bellerophon a golden bridle, which he used to tame Pegasus and defeat the Chimera.[1] In this mythical tale, the golden bridle gave man a combined means of wielding philosophical wisdom and human control over extraordinary entities. In Chapter 2, I explained the ways in which stem cell research is comprised of activities and technologies that are transformative and astonishing. Like the Greek hero Bellerophon, modern man, too, needs philosophical wisdom and local control – a golden bridle – to direct stem cell research.

The golden bridle offers an apt metaphor for what I believe are two different levels on which people tend to think about research ethics. Philosophers and others with theoretically inclined minds often like to discuss the ethics of scientific research at a very general, abstract level. For example, one may ask whether science is a human activity that is morally self-justifying, or whether it is valuable only in so far as it contributes to human flourishing. What makes the pursuit of scientific research morally good? Regarding stem cell research specifically, one may ask what moral values ought to guide its continuation, and what kind of limitations ought to constrain stem cell research in an ethically justified way? These are matters of philosophical research ethics. Philosophical research ethics is the stuff of philosophical wisdom, as represented by the golden nature of Athena's bridle.[2]

Others are inclined to talk about research ethics on a much more focused and practical level. Individuals such as research regulators and

---

[1] See my discussion of the Chimera myth in Chapter 1.
[2] The goddess Athena is closely associated with Western philosophy, and her symbol, the owl, is a favored mascot of many academic philosophy departments.

science practitioners may ask what ought to be required of scientists in order for their research proposals to be ethically permitted. Regarding stem cell scientists specifically, one might ask what it means for a particular basic or translational stem cell research project to be conducted in an ethical manner. The key questions here revolve not around which fundamental ethical grounds science should proceed upon, but rather in what ethical manner. The latter is a matter of practical research ethics. Practical research ethics is represented by the material bridle in the golden bridle metaphor – the practical means of exerting hands-on control over the earthly conduct of stem cell research.

We need to engage both of these levels in our thinking about the ethics of stem cell research. In this chapter, I explore further what I am calling *philosophical research ethics*. In Chapter 4 I take up the idea of practical research ethics. Ultimately, my aim in this and the following chapter is to advance two main points: that stem cell research offers us an opportunity to reexamine our understanding of research ethics at the philosophical and practical levels; and that some conflicts arising at the practical level are especially difficult because they are tied to uncertainties at the philosophical level.

## The Priority Question

Before I pursue these key issues, I wish to comment on some important preliminary matters. First, in contemplating the distinction between philosophical and practical research ethics, one might wonder which of these two levels is primary and which is derivative. Some theorists may respond that, clearly, philosophical research ethics must constitute the primary level, because it provides the reference points necessary to determine whether specific procedures at the practical ethics level are adequate for the task of research regulation. Philosophical research ethics, some may argue, supply the lofty ideals and core values that practical research ethics must then work to bring "down to earth."

I do not believe the answer is quite so obvious. For all we know, many of our philosophical ideals may derive from our reflections on real, practical life experiences. Philosophy is abstract; but we first need concrete examples from which to abstract our generalized ideas. On this view, our ideals do not descend down to us from Platonic heaven but are formed by the contours of the ground and ascend upward for us to debate their hazy shapes.

Those who would insist on the conceptual priority of philosophical research ethics also seem to have a valid point. Abstract ideals do appear to provide a guiding criterion by which we often make our everyday judgments and choices. For example, without the navigational star of first having a set of values at the philosophical research ethics level, there seems to be no way for us to answer the question "Why use this practical procedure for research approval and not some another?" Some might argue that the only way for us to justifiably choose one practical ethical procedure over another is by appealing to each one's capacity to realize a presupposed set of philosophical moral values. In light of these contraindicating considerations, my best guess is that the relationship between practical and philosophical research ethics is quite complex, and that each level informs and influences the other in a dynamic, bidirectional loop.[3]

It is worth acknowledging, however, that our traditional understanding of practical research ethics seems to have developed historically from philosophical values highlighted in seminal documents that comprise our international heritage of research ethics. One can infer from various ethical consensus statements, most notably the Nuremberg Code, the Declaration of Helsinki, and the Belmont Report, that there are abstract ethical values underwriting all biomedical research (which I soon discuss). From the philosophical values articulated in these documents arose a widely known set of recommendations and guidelines for ethical research. This historical (contingent) fact does not settle decisively the issue of conceptual priority between the two levels, but it does give us a place to begin our discussion. For expository convenience then, I begin with philosophical research ethics and proceed in the following chapter to practical research ethics.

## More Conceptual Dynamics

My second preliminary point is this. In addition to the dynamic relationship between philosophical and practical research ethics, there is

---

[3] By this I am not committing myself to a notion of reflective equilibrium first expounded by John Rawls and later extended to bioethical contexts by Norman Daniels. Reflective equilibrium is a coherentist theory of ethical and epsistemic justification (Daniels 1996; Rawls 1971). Personally, I favor an externalist foundationalist approach to ethical and epistemic justification. An exploration of these matters will take us far afield of our present concerns in this book, so I will have to save this discussion for another occasion.

another type of dynamic relationship we must bear in mind. This is the ongoing duel between consequentialist and deontological modes of ethical reasoning.

As discussed in Chapter 1, modern secular ethics can be characterized as a constant battle between (and within) consequentialist and deontological ethical camps. In various realms of normative bioethics, such as clinical ethics, research ethics, and policy decision making, a curious argumentative pattern seems to have evolved if one looks closely at how contentious issues are debated, such as health resource allocation and physician-assisted suicide. Positive consequentialist justifications for a particular course of action (e.g., restricting health care services for the elderly to increase resources for the young) must answer to one of two types of rebuttals: other consequentialist considerations that warn of alternative, negative effects of the action and deontological constraints that deny the proposed action on grounds that it violates people's moral rights (e.g., the elderly's right to needed health care). So consequentialism can be countered by consequentialist arguments for the other side and by deontological constraints. Likewise, positive deontological justifications for a course of action (e.g., allowing severely ill patients an autonomous option for physician-assisted suicide) must answer the same type of rebuttals: other deontological considerations (e.g., whether physician-assisted suicide countervails a doctor's duties to her patient) and consequentialist concerns that the proposed action may end up producing more overall harm than good, regardless of whether it is deontologically justified. So deontology can also be rebutted by other deontological constraints and by consequentialist arguments.

Modern secular ethics is much like a complex game of trumps, in which no one argumentative card is automatically privileged, be it of a consequentialist or deontological nature. To win an ethical debate, a contemporary bioethicist must convince others that her proposal does not irretrievably violate either consequentialist or deontological concerns that others may bring against it. If a proposal can reasonably withstand both types of rebuttals, then it may be said to be, at minimum, presumptively ethically permissible and, in some strong cases, even ethically obligatory.

One may pause here to ask why the natural law tradition in ethics cannot be invoked as an alternative framework for sorting through difficult normative ethical problems. To save space, I will address only the narrower question of whether the natural law tradition can help guide us in research ethics.

How would the natural law tradition answer the question "what makes research ethical?" According to natural law, the standard of rightness and wrongness is whether an act or state of affairs corresponds to God's plan for us and His divinely ordained natural order.[4] To put the matter succinctly, a natural law traditionalist must maintain that what is ethically right is that which God beneficently desires for us and the world.

Many religious individuals like to appeal to the natural law tradition to guide various aspects of their own personal lives. This I do not wish to deny. However, I believe applying this ethical approach to research ethics (and to other matters of public policy) is problematic for the following reasons.

First, the natural law tradition must posit the existence of God and His divine order, if natural law traditionalists are to issue ethical prescriptions for the rest of us that have any normative force. But then the question immediately becomes which conception of God (i.e., which world religion or which sect of Christianity) ought to serve as the background standard of value and whose exercise of reason is relevant for knowing what God's natural law demands of us? Thus the natural law tradition can be just as indeterminate as various secular ethics approaches, if not more so, because religious beliefs are matters of faith and not subject to standards of proof and evidence.

Second, if we take God completely out of the picture and rely solely on a person's own beliefs about the "natural order" of the world, we are no better off, because we can all challenge whether there is any normative wisdom contained in that person's exhortations to maintain the status quo – exhortations that must not simply collapse into secular deontological or consequentialist considerations, leaving natural law to do zero argumentative lifting.

This last point directs our attention to a general underlying problem for the natural law tradition, whether one posits the existence of God. The problem lies in the natural law tradition's propensity to elevate the status quo to an ethically authoritative level. Unfortunately, as we have seen in the previous two chapters, science has a vexing tendency to disrupt our tidy conceptual categories and traditional practices – categories and practices that comprise the very status quo that is so beloved by natural law traditionalists. The natural law tradition relies on the assumption that our important conceptual categories and practices can remain stable. But if our categories and understandings of how the world is

---

[4] See my discussion of the natural law tradition in ethics in Chapter 1.

ordered are malleable as the result of new human conditions and practices, then the natural law tradition loses the fixed points necessary to
instruct us on how to act.

Expanding on this last point, I suggest that the natural law tradition
is not well suited to answer the question "what makes research ethical?"
at either the philosophical or practical level. In order for natural law to
provide guidance for research, many, if not most, scientific techniques
would have to be abandoned. That is, according to the implicit norms
of the natural law tradition, scientists must only passively observe and
record the "natural order" of the world; they must never disrupt this
order during their act of observation. However, stem cell science – like
all other forms of biomedical research and technological advancement –
violates this observation constraint. In the process of studying how stem
cells function, for example, researchers must cultivate or form new biological entities (e.g., pluripotent stem cells or chimeric animals) that
do not have obvious analogues in the developed human body or in the
animal kingdom. The "unnatural" is an anathema for the natural law tradition in ethics. But all branches of the modern biological sciences must
proceed through the performance of unnatural acts.

Despite all its indeterminacies, modern secular ethics at least allows
for the possibility that unnatural acts may be ethically permissible. In
some cases, unnatural acts could even be ethically obligatory, such as
doctors' providing chemotherapy or blood transfusions for gravely ill
patients. In the case of blood stem cell transplantation for childhood leukemia, for example, this intervention transforms pediatric patients into
human-to-human chimeras: that is, the patient's blood system is recon-
stituted using hematopoetic stem cells from a donor source, sometimes
of the opposite sex, thereby rendering that patient's blood cells forever
genetically distinct from the rest of his somatic cells.

If unnatural acts are an ineliminable part of science and biomedical
research, then research ethics must provide room for the performance
of these unnatural acts. Ultimately, the important distinction for research
ethics is not between the natural and the unnatural; rather, it is between
the ethically unnatural and the unethically unnatural.

Critics may respond that, without the eternal dictates of natural law,
all we are left with is the "thin gruel" of modern secular ethics – thin
because we would be left with no substantive conception of the Good
for persons, only an indeterminate game of trumps. I disagree with this
dire diagnosis, because I believe that the value of personal autonomy
(to take one example) constitutes one of the central components of our

leading a good life. Not only is personal autonomy an essential element of a flourishing existence, but its exercise is instrumentally crucial for directing each person toward his or her own specific good. On this view, there exists not a *single* Good for all persons, but rather *plural goods* that the exercise of personal autonomy helps to identify and match up to each unique individual.[5]

What is important to realize here is that – unlike the eternal dictates of the natural law tradition – the core ethical values underlying philosophical research ethics are sufficiently general and flexible to remain relevant in an ever-changing world. All human beings are born dependent and usually die in a similar state of dependence. From the beginning of life to the end, we remain physically, psychologically, and socially vulnerable to harm. Human beings also have basic rights and the capacity to exercise these rights. These universal truths make the core values of philosophical research ethics always pertinent, always applicable, regardless of whether we live in a modern world with categories constantly in flux due to new scientific and technical advancements. With these preliminary comments out of the way, I now wish to discuss the core values underlying scientific research.

## Philosophical Research Ethics

Biomedical research is an activity that is heavily tilted toward a consequentialist mode of evaluation. Although some defenders of science may advance the liberal nonconsequentialist point that scientists have a right to seek knowledge (Robertson 1978), by and large research is a goal-oriented activity. After all, a scientist can exercise her right to pursue knowledge, but do so poorly, using the wrong methodology. What separates scientifically good research from scientifically bad research is whether the methods a scientist uses can deliver an increase in generalizable understanding, not whether she has exercised her right to pursue knowledge. Although we may hope that a scientist conducts her research voluntarily (and thus consciously exercises her right to pursue knowledge), what really matters from the standpoint of scientific evaluation is whether her research reveals truths.

But while the ultimate aim of research is to expand knowledge, the moral worth of research derives not from the intrinsic value of new

---

[5] John Stuart Mill defends a view of human flourishing very similar to this in his works *On Liberty* (1859) and *The Subjection of Women* (1869).

knowledge, but from the ways in which that knowledge may be used to improve the human condition and protect our vulnerabilities. It is through its capacity to grant empowering knowledge that the conduct of research gains a moral character. The pursuit of knowledge simply for knowledge's sake is not itself a moral endeavor; rather, it is a perfectionist value. Only when new knowledge impacts human welfare does it become interesting from a moral point of view and not simply from the epistemic standpoint of perfecting humankind's collective system of beliefs.

All morally relevant scientific research aims to produce consequential gains in knowledge that may positively impact human well-being in some way or another. In opposition to this consequentialist justification for scientific research are countervailing consequentialist arguments to the effect that scientific research produces on balance more dystopian uses of new knowledge than not. I wish to set such countervailing consequentialist rebuttals aside for the moment and concentrate on the tension between proscience moral consequentialism and deontology.

There are other moral standards that bear on science besides the promotion of human welfare–contributing knowledge. To illustrate, consider the following counterfactual scenario. If promoting knowledge were the sole moral standard for science, then there ought to be no problem in principle for scientists to treat human subjects the same way they treat animal subjects – as mere instruments for scientific studies. In animal experimentation, scientists breed animals to have certain medically relevant characteristics (e.g., liver deficiencies) or they produce controlled injuries in animals (e.g., strokes or myocardial ischemia), after which researchers try to ameliorate these humanlike ailments in a study.[6] In animal research, scientists do not need to ask animals for their permission, nor do they need to consider how the burdens of research will be distributed amongst the animals. If human subjects research were conducted in the same manner (perhaps by using small populations of unlucky persons against their will), then science might proceed much faster toward socially important advances, such as a cure for HIV/AIDS or cancer.

Should we, for the sake of maximal efficiency, allow human subjects research to be conducted no differently from animal research? Obviously not. As the preceding counterfactual is meant to reveal, advancing research is important, but there are other moral values at stake for science. Primary among these values is the moral requirement that we treat all

---

[6] I offer here a simplified account of animal research in order to make my point. I explore in Chapters 5 and 6 the many complex issues surrounding animal research.

human research subjects as persons deserving of respect. Thus, although science is goal oriented and measured against results-driven standards of success and although it is (largely) morally justified on consequentialist grounds, it is at the same time constrained by deontological limitations on what can be done to human beings in the pursuit of knowledge.

As a product of modernity, philosophical research ethics is a dynamic and uncertain field of inquiry. Standing at opposite ends are our two starting points. The moral value of scientific research is largely consequentialist. Human protections are largely deontological. The net result of this duality is that we are faced with the task of having to balance two very different standards of ethics against one other. *Balance* is the right term here, for we cannot favor the one by completely forsaking the other. Promoting rapid advances in knowledge can perhaps be maximally achieved if we ignore human protections for the unlucky few called into experimentation. The surest way to protect human subjects from being harmed in a study is to forbid human research altogether, because all such research involves some level of attendant risk, however minimal. Neither of these extreme positions is ethically desirable. The right approach must lie somewhere in the middle. Thus, at the heart of philosophical research ethics is a constant tension between the consequentialist engine of science and the deontological brakes of human subject protections.

This need to balance consequentialist and deontological considerations is apparent in historically significant documents that have helped shape our understanding of research ethics today. Consider three prominent examples: the Nuremberg Code, the Declaration of Helsinki, and the Belmont Report.[7] Although none of these documents can be said to

---

7 The Nuremberg Code (1946–9) is a list of ten ethical standards for human experimentation that arose from the Nuremberg War Crime Trials at the end of World War II. Originally appearing as a subsection of the trial proceedings entitled "Permissible Medical Experiments," the Nuremberg Code (as it later came to be known) set forth ethical standards against which physicians and scientists who conducted medical experiments on concentration camp prisoners were judged. The Nuremberg Code remained a sealed court document for a period of time before it was made publicly available, after which it became the template of many later codes of research ethics.

The Declaration of Helsinki (1964) was adopted by the General Assembly of the World Medical Association to guide medical doctors in the ethical conduct of human experimentation. To date, it has undergone six substantial revisions (most recently in 2008) and has evolved from 11 original paragraphs to 35. With each iteration, the declaration has departed further from the Nuremberg Code by adding considerations not addressed in the latter. For instance, the declaration now addresses (albeit briefly) vulnerable research populations, surrogate consent, the need for ethical review committees,

have invented the core values at work in philosophical research ethics, each offers an interpretation of what these core values are and how they relate to the ethical conduct of research. Whether their implied interpretations of these values are philosophically sound is a topic for discussion later. Let us examine the fundamental values defended in these documents before we critique their apparent theoretical interpretations and presumptions.

Despite their individual differences, the Nuremburg Code, the Declaration of Helsinki, and the Belmont Report together identify (implicitly and explicitly) important values underlying the ethical conduct of research. These values should be seen as additional ethical considerations to be weighed alongside the consequentialist moral value of welfare-impacting scientific research.[8]

## Scientific Integrity

Scientific integrity is a multifaceted concept that bears high instrumental and high ethical value. The word *integrity* comes from the Latin

---

the use of placebos in research, the use of identifiable human material and data, and medical innovation outside of clinical trials. With each addition, the declaration has become more and more controversial, with some regulatory bodies, such the European Commission, recognizing only earlier versions of the declaration, and others, such as the FDA and the NIH, eliminating all reference to it in their training programs. For these reasons, I base my analyses in this chapter on earlier, more widely influential versions of the declaration.

The Belmont Report (1979) was created by the U.S. National Commission for the Protection of Human Subjects of Biomedical and Behavioral Research. Officially entitled "Ethical Principles and Guidelines for the Protection of Human Subjects of Research," the Belmont Report (as it is now widely called) articulated fundamental ethical principles for all human subjects research.

[8] Curiously, only the Nuremberg Code explicitly mentions the requirement that scientific research "should be such as to yield fruitful results *for the good of society*" (1946–9, 181, emphasis mine). In the Belmont Report, this social-benefit requirement appears to be quietly subsumed under the principle of beneficence. I assume the Declaration of Helsinki simply accepts this requirement implicitly.

This relative lack of attention to the social-benefit requirement of scientific research in these documents is unfortunate. As I argue in the preceding text, the consequentialist moral justification of science is an absolutely crucial element of philosophical research ethics. Without it there would be no moral counterweight to the deontological constraints of human protections, and therefore no real complexity to the possible debates in philosophical research ethics. Furthermore, a practical implication of omitting this requirement is that it would be very difficult to justify ever conducting first-in-human clinical trials or any other early stage human experimentation (such as phase I drug safety studies using healthy volunteers) where there is little or no possibility of direct benefit for research subjects. It would be irrational to allow human subjects to be exposed to such risks without any counterbalancing possibility of social benefit deriving from the research.

*integritas*, meaning "wholeness" or "completeness." When viewed from one angle, scientific integrity appears to be solely a technical demand for conducting scientific investigations competently, using sound scientific methodologies. For example, it is not enough merely to desire that one's experiment reveal the truth; the experiment must be designed rigorously to address a hypothesis-driven question using statistically valid methods. And it must be conducted by scientifically qualified personnel, not simply those who are deeply curious.

On this first interpretation, scientific integrity is an ideal of scientific completeness or soundness. Scientific integrity in this sense is captured through statements in the Nuremberg Code asserting that an experiment "should be so designed and based on the results of animal experimentation and a knowledge of the natural history of the disease or other problem under study that the anticipated results will justify the performance of the experiment" and that "the experiment should be conducted only by qualified persons" (Nuremberg Code 1946–9). The Declaration of Helsinki states similarly that "[m]edical research involving human subjects must conform to generally accepted scientific principles, be based on a thorough knowledge of the scientific literature, other relevant sources of information, and on an adequate laboratory and, where appropriate, animal experimentation." Also, "[m]edical research involving human subjects should be conducted only by scientifically qualified persons and under the supervision of a clinically competent medical person" (World Medical Association 1964). Scientific integrity in this first sense is essentially a reminder that science must be performed precisely and skillfully, and that it must aim to contribute to an ongoing narrative of the scientific problem at hand. An experiment must never be sloppy, random, or unnecessary in nature.

This is all well and good, one may argue, but what does scientific integrity in this technical sense have to do with ethics? Seen from a different angle, the same demands of technical scientific integrity carry considerable moral weight. For one thing, if a scientific experiment is poorly designed or performed in a way that destroys its likelihood of unveiling truths, then it immediately loses its moral consequentialist justification (i.e., its positive moral status as a welfare-enhancing knowledge promoter). Furthermore, a lack of scientific integrity in the technical sense results in a waste of resources (be they economic, material, or animal) and in the needless exposure of human subjects to risk. For these reasons, it is a mistake to think that science and ethics are two entirely separate domains of concern, because often what first appears to be a simple scientific issue turns out – through a Gestalt shift in perspective – to be a matter of deep ethical significance and vice versa.

My point here about the hazy line between scientific and ethical concerns can be further illuminated if readers recall my discussion in Chapter 2 about the need to continue iPS cell and hES cell research together. Critical patient safety issues hang in the balance of sorting through what may initially appear to be just "technical questions" about their biological equivalence and the best methods to characterize and process their direct derivatives. Issues such as these are equally scientific and ethical.

The preceding analysis places the moral value of scientific integrity squarely in the consequentialists' camp. On this approach, technical scientific integrity is morally relevant because it is needed to produce the socially beneficial results demanded by the consequentialist moral justification of science. But there exists another, nonconsequential-ist interpretation of the moral relevance of scientific integrity. On this interpretation, scientific integrity is morally valuable because it relates to a scientist's duty to be a spokesperson for truth. That is, a scientist must not only seek the truth using sound, empirically verifiable methods, but she also must accept her conclusions, however inconvenient they may be politically, commercially, or ideologically. Furthermore, she must communicate her conclusions truthfully and without hype to the public, funders, publishers, and the greater scientific community.[9] In this sense, scientific integrity is an ideal, not just for the process of conducting sci-ence, but for the scientist – a type of personal wholeness between her scientific commitments and her actions. Here, scientific integrity might be viewed as a virtue of character, along the lines of certain virtue eth-ics theories, or as part of a larger deontological duty to live one's life in accordance with the truth. In either case, this second sense of scientific integrity falls outside the consequentialists' camp.

All three of these aspects of scientific integrity are important – the technical, the morally consequential, and the obligations of truthful-ness – for they intertwine to form a sturdy canvas upon which the pri-mary colors of beneficence, respect for persons, and justice are layered, creating a full and weighty portrait of philosophical research ethics.

---

[9] This sense of scientific integrity as truthfulness of the scientist did not appear in the Declaration of Helsinki until later versions. "In publication of the results of research, the investigators are obliged to preserve the accuracy of the results. Negative as well as positive results should be published or otherwise publicly available" (World Medical Association 1964).

Without first having the mixed fabric of scientific integrity before us, there would be no reason for us to entertain questions about where the other moral values ought to be placed on this canvas, how they should relate to one another, or their levels of intensity. Without scientific integrity, there would be no reason to proceed to discussions about the role of beneficence, respect for persons, and justice in scientific research.

## Beneficence

Beneficence is a key moral value that bears directly on science. But it is a complex concept, and it deserves to be unpacked before we discuss its role in philosophical research ethics and stem cell research. Beneficence is the moral obligation to contribute to the welfare of others. Conceptually, the duty of beneficence is more stringent than the duty of nonmaleficence (the duty to do no harm).[10] Whereas nonmaleficence obligates an individual simply to refrain from harming others, beneficence calls upon her to perform positive actions to promote others' welfare. It is precisely this requirement for positive action that makes the duty of beneficence much more demanding. At the end of the day, a person can ask herself whether she has adequately satisfied her duty of nonmaleficence. If she has not caused anyone harm, then she can confidently say her duty has been fulfilled. Beneficence, however, is much more open-ended, for a person can also ask herself at the end of the day whether she has satisfied this duty, and the answer may not be so clear. She could possess a nagging doubt as to whether she has done all she can to promote others' welfare or whether she has fallen short of fully satisfying this duty.

Because of this nagging open-endedness, some theorists have insisted on setting a limit on the duty of beneficence to make it more achievable. Deontologists typically try to draw a distinction between obligatory beneficence and supererogatory beneficence (i.e., the actual duty of beneficence versus beneficence that goes beyond the call of duty). The challenge, however, is how to draw this distinction nonarbitrarily. For example, we cannot simply mark out a line based on what we are

---

[10] Nonmaleficence is one of the primary moral duties of a physician in a clinical care context. (*Primum non nocere*, "First do no harm.") However, in a research context, the duty of nonmaleficence is not usually believed to be essential and may make human subjects research ethically untenable insofar as the exposure of persons to harm is an ineliminable part of biomedical research. Research-related harms cannot be ruled out as a practical matter of fact, but instead must be balanced against potential benefits, as the duty of beneficence described in this section attempts to do.

habitually willing and unwilling to do for others. In an effort to make the duty of beneficence more "livable," we cannot simply privilege (as we are usually apt to do) our special relations and our limited empathy for faraway strangers, at least not without further philosophical defense.

In order to avoid explaining the deontologists' boundary between duty and the supererogatory, some may argue that beneficence is a moral value that can also be grounded in consequentialism, not just deontology. Promoting the welfare of others is one of the central features of many forms of consequentialism, particularly a subset known as *utilitarianism*. Utilitarianism maintains that the good must always be maximized through one's choice of alternative actions. However, by grounding beneficence in consequentialism, we are brought right back to our old problem. One of the chief critiques of consequentialism, especially utilitarianism, is that it demands precisely the kind of unlimited beneficence that nagged us earlier. Critics have argued that the consequentialist duty to maximize others' benefits would be too morally demanding if we were to accept it and that it would turn us each into obsessive utility-maximizers with no recognizable lives or projects to call our own (Williams 1973).

In response, consequentialists might argue that the demands of beneficence could be bounded by additional consequentialist concerns about the damage that unlimited beneficence could have on our own plans of life. But this consolation seems to fall far short of a satisfactory answer, because the demands of beneficence can still go quite a long way toward driving people close to exhaustion before it is reigned in by its expanding negative personal consequences. The demands of beneficence implied by consequentialism would make monks out of each of us, austere and stripped of our own personal attachments.

Regardless of whether the obligation of beneficence is understood deontologically (as bounded with unexplained borders) or consequentially (as potentially exhausting and life altering), beneficence remains a very important moral value in the conduct of science. Beneficence on the part of scientists can be directed toward society at large or to the individuals participating in research.[11] We have already seen in the preceding

---

[11] The Belmont Report recognizes the latter of these two directions (beneficence directed toward individuals) but not the former (beneficence directed toward society). Curiously, however, the report recognizes an opposite obligation of beneficence on the part of society at large toward *"the entire enterprise of research"* (Department of Health, Education and Welfare 1979, emphasis mine). "In the case of scientific research in general, members of the larger society are obligated to recognize the longer term benefits and risks that may result from the improvement of knowledge and from the development of novel medical, psychotherapeutic, and social procedures."

text how beneficence in the first sense – benefit to society – is implicit in the consequentialist moral justification of science. When beneficence is aimed at individual human research subjects, it obligates researchers and science regulators to try to minimize potential harms and maximize potential benefits for study volunteers. As the Belmont Report states, "In the case of particular projects, investigators and members of their institutions are obliged to give forethought to the maximization of benefits and the reduction of risk that might occur from the research investigation" (Department of Health, Education and Welfare 1979).

At this point, our nagging doubts about the limits of beneficence creep back into the discussion. What does it mean for science to fulfill its social obligation of beneficence? For example, how directly should research results impact human welfare for science to be morally justified? And can the promise of social benefit be fulfilled simply through the generation of (expensive) commercial medical products and services, or does social benefit have to be realized in some other, more broadly accessible form? These are crucial and difficult philosophical questions for stem cell research.

With respect to beneficence directed at human research subjects, we may ask what science practitioners and regulators are obligated to do and how far they must go to meet their obligations. The Nuremberg Code states that researchers should avoid any *unnecessary* physical and mental suffering and injury, and that the degree of risk involved in a study must never exceed its humanitarian importance. Similarly, the Declaration of Helsinki recommends that research should only be carried out if the importance of the research goal outweighs the risks to human subjects. The Belmont Report provides a bit more guidance than the others by stating that researchers and regulators must consider many different types of risks and benefits. Risks to the subject can be physical, psychological, legal, social, and economic. Benefits to the subject may be physical and psychological. Benefits can also include broader gains for society and for science. The Belmont Report, however, is silent on the issue of how far science practitioners and regulators ought to go to minimize the aforementioned harms and maximize the benefits; its only recommendation on this score is that the overall risk-benefit ratio for research must be shown to be reasonable. But how, we may ask, is it conceptually possible to balance such varied risks and benefits? Are there any other beneficent actions required of scientists and regulators besides striving for reasonable risk-benefit ratios? We return to these philosophical questions in Chapter 7.

*Respect for Persons*

"Respect for persons" is perhaps the most well-known of all the research-related moral values. Typically this requirement is understood to entail that human subjects must give their informed consent if they are to be used in scientific research. The Nuremberg Code begins with the stark statement that "[t]he voluntary consent of the human subject is absolutely essential." The Declaration of Helsinki states that "subjects must be volunteers and informed participants in the research project." To respect persons in this manner is to honor their right to make decisions over their own lives and bodies. This right is normally referred to as the right to personal autonomy or the right to self-determination.[12]

Traditionally, autonomy theorists have advanced deeply rationalistic conceptions of what it means to act autonomously. For example, some philosophers have argued that all autonomous actions arise from a person's successful performance of certain mental operations, such as higher-order desiring and critical self-evaluation (Dworkin 1970; Frankfurt 1971). However, there is no need to remain wedded to these early accounts nor do we need to accept the rugged individualism that these rationalist conceptions imply. I believe a more philosophically defensible conception of personal autonomy would define self-determination in terms of a person's acting on her authentic values, be they communal values, cultural values, or self-interested prudential values (Hyun 2001).[13] This more expansive approach to understanding autonomy is consistent with the medical profession's current tendency to allow variable degrees of patient involvement in the informed consent

---

[12] Contemporary philosophers typically view personal autonomy as a component of individual well-being. In this sense, it should be distinguished from the concept of moral autonomy, which is essentially a doctrine about the nature of morality (Raz 1986). Personal autonomy concerns the capability of persons to choose the course of their own lives, and it is directly contrasted with paternalism. It is only very indirectly related to the Kantian idea that the basis of morality consists of rational, self-legislated, and universalizable maxims (Kant 1785). These two forms of autonomy need not coincide, for individuals can pursue immoral ends without necessarily losing their personal autonomy; however, no person can remain morally autonomous while acting immorally. To summarize, moral autonomy – whether in the Kantian or other versions – is a specific metaethical position, while personal autonomy is broader and may be included as one element in numerous, possibly even opposing, moral doctrines.

[13] Gary Watson (1975) agrees that what is of central importance for autonomy is that a person act in accordance with her values. Other theoretical maneuvers, such as Dworkin's and Frankfurt's notions of higher-order desiring, are extraneous for an adequate conception of individual autonomy. As Watson succinctly explains, a person acts autonomously only when her "valuational system" coincides with her "motivational system."

process and over the range of medical alternatives, as directed by the patient's values (Hyun 2002).

Returning to the context of research ethics, it should be pointed out that honoring autonomous decision making through informed consent is but one interpretation (albeit a very important one) of what it means to respect persons in the course of scientific investigation. According to the Belmont Report and the Declaration of Helsinki, respect for persons also entails that researchers must not take unfair advantage of individuals lacking autonomy, such as young children and decisionally incapacitated adults. Neither must researchers exploit individuals with diminished autonomy who are susceptible to undue social pressures to participate in research, such as prisoners, the poor, and the gravely ill. In this regard, respect for persons is not simply a restatement of the deontological duty to recognize personal autonomy – it is much broader than this. It includes respecting individuals who have little or no autonomy.

Philosophical questions swirl around what it means to respect persons, either as autonomous decision makers (with whom others might disagree about what is best for them) or as individuals with diminished or no autonomy (whom we are obligated to treat appropriately). How can respect for persons encompass such disparate types of individuals? That is, how can respect for persons entail respect for autonomous decision making and yet also apply to individuals who lack autonomy, either partially or fully? To sort through these questions, we should consider separately the two constitutive components of respect for persons.

The notion of "respect" comes to us from the Latin *respectus*, meaning "to look back." The etymology of respect is especially illuminating when one considers how the deontological constraint of respect for persons is typically contrasted with consequentialist modes of ethical evaluation. Recall that, according to consequentialism, the appropriate moral response to any object of intrinsic moral value is to promote it, either in number, duration, intensity, and the like. According to deontology, in contrast, the appropriate response to an object of intrinsic moral value is respect. The deontologist does not look forward like the consequentialist by asking herself how she ought to promote a thing of value; rather, she "looks back" and honors that which is morally valuable by getting out of the way, by honoring it with the freedom to be as it were.

In research, we are obligated to respect all human subjects as persons. The word *person* comes from the Latin *persona*, which means "a character in a drama, or a mask worn in a drama." Traditionally, philosophers have taken the concept of a person to be broader than the concept of a human being, because, conceivably, some nonhumans (perhaps intelligent aliens or thinking computers) could have the necessary attributes of personhood, or, alternatively, a single human being could host more than one person (as appears to be the case with multiple personality disorder). Philosophers usually identify certain highly intellectual psychological characteristics, such as critical self-awareness or rationality and the capacity for higher-order desires (i.e., the desire *to desire X*) as the touchstones of personhood (Frankfurt 1971). On this view, persons are essentially defined in cognitivist, autonomy-focused terms, not biological or physical terms as implied by the category of human being.

Unfortunately, such a deeply rationalist approach to personhood poses serious problems if we want to include children and decisionally incapacitated adults under our obligation to respect persons during the course of scientific research. As suggested by the Declaration of Helsinki and the Belmont Report, our duty to respect human subjects as persons extends to research studies involving pediatric patients and seniors with dementia. This is not an issue that can simply be resolved through surrogate consent, for what others (e.g., parents, caretakers, and the like) are obliged to do in providing surrogate consent is likewise to treat their dependent as a person deserving of respect. Thus we are still faced with the duty to respect as persons potential research subjects who would otherwise fail to meet many philosophers' highly cognitivist requirements for personhood.

An alternative approach to defining personhood would be to take a nonessentialist view that resists identifying a single property or a very narrowly defined cluster of properties as constitutive of what it means to be a person. Rather, a person could be defined as a bundle of characteristics, with no single one of these characteristics as being absolutely essential for personhood. A nonessentialist approach would perhaps resolve the philosophical paradox presented in trying to reconcile traditional intellectualist models of personhood with the much more capacious respect-for-persons requirement underscored by the Declaration of Helsinki and Belmont Report.

### Justice
Justice is another deontological value that bears on the conduct of science. In its most generic sense, the concept of justice requires impartially that persons receive what is owed to them. Applied to the area of criminal wrongdoing, for instance, criminal justice demands that persons be punished in proportion to their crimes. Rectificatory justice calls for the

compensation for personal losses due to injury or a breach of contract. For our purposes, the conception of justice relevant for research ethics is *distributive justice*, which involves the impartial distribution of burdens and benefits among individuals or groups.

Distributive justice in research requires that burdens and benefits be fairly distributed, during the course of research among human subjects and later when research results become available to broader segments of society. For example, the Belmont Report states that human subjects must be fairly selected to volunteer for research, not systematically chosen from vulnerable populations because they are easy to manipulate. Nor should subjects be selected from groups unlikely to benefit from later applications of the research (Department of Health, Education and Welfare 1979). Likewise, the Declaration of Helsinki states that "[m]edical research is only justified if there is a reasonable likelihood that the populations in which the research is carried out stand to benefit from the results of the research" (World Medical Association 1964).

Distributive justice, like respect for persons, is a deontological constraint on the consequentialist enterprise of scientific research. The need for such a constraint was highlighted by historical atrocities in research, such as the Willowbrook State School hepatitis study and the Tuskegee Syphilis Study, both conducted by U.S. government agencies and both lacking fair selection of subjects (in addition to lacking informed consent and reasonable risk-benefit ratios). These and many other cases like them revealed the need to take justice very seriously in defining the ethical requirements for research.

However, as with the other moral values discussed in this chapter, important theoretical issues remain to be clarified. Although most observers will readily admit that the burdens and benefits of research ought to be distributed fairly, it is not so apparent exactly which distributive principle ought to guide this ideal. There are several different distributive principles of justice from which a theorist might choose. One may, for example, argue that the burdens and benefits ought to be distributed among study participants by lottery (e.g., random assignment to experimental and control groups), by level of personal contribution (e.g., compensation for time, effort, and inconvenience), or according to free-market exchanges (e.g., monetary incentives for research participation).

None of the historically significant research ethics consensus documents offers ways to clarify these important details. But it is precisely these details that matter most when thinking about how justice actually ought to factor into the conduct of scientific research. With respect to the broader social impact of stem cell research, for example, one can question whether the just distribution of stem cell–based therapies should be determined solely by free-market exchanges or whether special concessions need to be made for patients with intractable conditions based on their health needs. It is one thing merely to note that justice has a role in the ethical conduct of science; it is another thing entirely – a far more difficult and important task – to defend which distributive principle of justice ought to guide the sharing of research benefits and burdens among study participants and among larger segments of society.

In summary, there are four main moral values at work in philosophical research ethics. Scientific integrity is first and foremost on the list, for without it there is no need to balance considerations regarding the other three values: beneficence, respect for persons, and justice. When upheld in concert, these four values are together supposed to constitute a response to the theoretical question "what make research ethical?"

## Balancing and the Incommensurability Problem

If ethical research is supposed to weigh each of these values against one another, then a key philosophical question for us to consider is how such a balancing act is possible. Balancing disparate values, such as beneficence and respect for persons, presupposes that there is a single scale upon which these different values can be perched and weighed. But this raises a philosophical conundrum. If these four core values are fundamental and distinct from one another, with none being reducible to any of the others, then we have, by definition, a problem of *incommensurability*. Two or more values (or the bearers of values) are incommensurable when there is no single common unit of value by which they can all be measured (Chang 1997). The incommensurability problem can be stated as follows: if two or more values are incommensurable – that is, if they cannot be compared to one another in reference to a common unit of value – then their incommensurability precludes the possibility of there being a justified choice among them.[14] With respect to the four core moral values of philosophical research ethics, then, the threat of their incommensurability would preclude the possibility of there being a justifiable way to balance each against the others. I believe

---

[14] Some philosophers have argued that incommensurable goods can still be compared – that incommensurability does not necessarily entail *incomparability* (Chang 1997). I critique this position in Chapter 7.

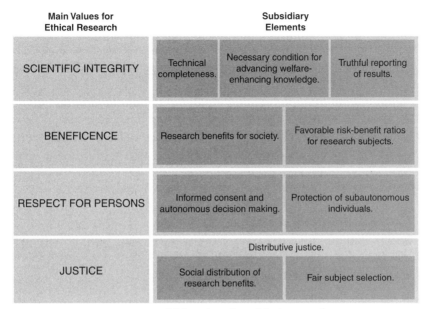

FIGURE 3.1. Main values for ethical research.

the incommensurability problem and the force of its implications have been insufficiently appreciated by other theorists working in stem cell research ethics.

I return to the incommensurability problem in Chapter 7, but for now I wish to acknowledge one possible way to reduce (although not eliminate) its damage. To do this, we may point out that there is significant overlap among many of the main values for ethical research. Importantly, as I argued previously, each of these four core values is analyzable in further specified ways. For example, we have already seen that scientific integrity and beneficence each have different subsidiary elements relating to their scope and direction of applicability (see Figure 3.1). The same holds true for respect for persons and justice.

It is important to recognize that, when the four main values interact, they do so at the sublevel of their subsidiary elements. The incommensurability problem can be reduced (although not eliminated completely) if some of these elements can be shown to overlap to a significant degree. For example, both respect for persons and justice are very closely related regarding the former's required protection of subautonomous (socially and psychologically vulnerable) individuals and the latter's condition for fair subject selection. Likewise, beneficence and justice are closely related in their demand that research must benefit society beyond those who are directly involved in the study. Nonsupererogatory (dutiful) beneficence renders the aim of social benefit a morally binding one. Principles of distributive justice make the social distribution of research benefits similarly morally binding, because to say that a segment of society is due certain research benefits is to say that these individuals have a justice claim on that which is rightfully owed to them.

This manner of confronting the incommensurability problem is not a reductionist strategy, because I am not claiming that any one of the main moral values underwriting science is wholly equivalent to any other. Only some of the values' subsidiary elements overlap, not all. There are limits to this unifying strategy. Incompatibilities among core moral values do not disappear entirely, and we are still forced to deal with a level of incommensurability in the end.

## Conclusion

Our focus in this chapter on philosophical research ethics – understood as a separate but related sphere hovering above our more practical interest in research ethics – reveals three often-overlooked points. The first is that the core moral values of philosophical research ethics tend to align along either consequentialist or nonconsequentialist modes of ethical reasoning. Because of their fundamentally different ethical alignments, questions regarding how best to balance the values of scientific integrity, beneficence, respect for persons, and justice often produce indeterminate answers. For example, we saw that the moral justification for science rests on the consequential promise of social benefit, while the constraints placed on scientific investigation are grounded largely on nonconsequentialist human subjects protections. In times of conflict, which should override the other? What about first-in-human clinical trials, where the tensions between potential social benefits (in the form of expanding scientific knowledge) and the unknown risks to human subjects are especially contentious? The answers are far from clear. This should come as no surprise to philosophers, because we are being asked to compare in some meaningful way the normative dictates of two opposite modes of moral evaluation.

Compounding this first difficulty is what I have called the incommensurability problem. The very idea that we can strike a rightful balance among the four core values of philosophical research ethics presupposes that these values are commensurable on a common scale of evaluation.

But this presupposition flies in the face of the simultaneous belief that none of these values is merely reducible to the others – that they are each fundamentally different values. Thus arises the incommensurability problem.

Finally, it should be observed that, among the four core values of research ethics, the duties of social beneficence and distributive justice ought to be explored much further. Within the context of scientific research, there are still open questions involving (1) *what* counts as a relevant social benefit, (2) *who* bears the duty of providing and distributing the social benefits of science, (3) *to whom* such benefits are owed, and (4) *how far* this duty extends (understood here as an *actual duty* and not some supererogatory provision of benefits). The questions of "what," "who," "to whom," and "how far" are crucial and have not been adequately addressed in the area of stem cell research.

This is unfortunate because so much of the political rhetoric supporting stem cell research in the United States and in many other countries has been built vaguely upon the great future promise of stem cell research. For example, Harold Varmus, then Director of the U.S. National Institutes of Health (NIH), famously testified before a Senate appropriations subcommittee that federal funding for hES cell research should go forward because of the field's great promise for medical advancements (Varmus 1999).

What promissory statements such as these tend to gloss over are the all-important specifics of "what," "who," "to whom," and "how far." For example, we saw in Chapter 2 that the advancement of basic stem cell science and its clinical translation is an extremely collaborative enterprise involving basic scientists, clinicians, bioengineers, study sponsors, manufacturers, cell and tissue repositories, and many other intermediaries. If anyone is to bear the moral duty of social beneficence, then each one of these parties must carry their own proportionate share of it. But what this actually means in real practical and philosophical terms I have little idea. Furthermore, to whom is this duty owed? The general notion of social benefit fails to capture the real-world point that society is not all of one piece but rather is comprised of many different stakeholders who have greater or lesser moral claims to the benefits in question. What counts as a social benefit borne out of stem cell research? And how far must the duty-bound go to fulfill their obligations of social beneficence? It is difficult to know which of these hard questions to tackle first, for each one seems to presuppose that the others have been answered in some preliminary way. There is much work for practical and theoretical bioethicists to sort through in just this one corner of philosophical research ethics.

In summary, the golden bridle of philosophical research ethics turns out to be an elusive and underdeveloped area of bioethics. Philosophical probing of these values and their interrelationships seems to raise more questions than answers. But such is the nature of philosophical investigation. The important point is that we discover through this process which questions are especially worth asking and pursuing.

Practical research ethics as it relates to stem cell research is also in need of further refinement, particularly where it deals with types of research not well suited to traditional regulatory approaches. Historically speaking, practical research ethics can be characterized as an institutionally mandated minimum floor of human protections below which consequentially driven science may never dip. Unlike philosophical research ethics – which concerns open-ended issues such as how far our obligations take us, who has these obligations, and who is owed benefits and why – practical research ethics deals with defining thresholds for ethically permissible research and guarding these thresholds. In Chapter 4 we turn to practical research ethics and explore the adequacy of these thresholds against the rising tides of stem cell research.

# 4

## The Golden Bridle II

### *Practical Research Ethics*

The regulation of stem cell research in the United States is comprised of a combination of decades-old federal human subjects protections plus a set of stem cell research–specific ethical standards voluntarily adopted by institutions since 2005.[1] In this chapter I trace over the main contours of these two components, acknowledging along the way new questions that emerge concerning the limits of these approaches to overseeing the stem cell field.

### From Belmont Principles to Federal Regulation

In the United States there is a close historical connection between the philosophical ethical principles outlined in the Belmont Report and the federal regulation of human subjects research. Widespread public revelations of exploitive scientific studies using vulnerable populations, such as the Tuskegee Syphilis Study and the Willowbrook State School hepatitis study, led the U.S. Senate to pass the National Research Act of 1974. This act achieved two very important results. First, it established the requirement that anyone applying for a federal grant to support research using human subjects must have their study proposals reviewed by an independent local committee known as an Institutional Review Board (IRB), which is responsible for protecting the rights and interests

---

[1] In addition to these general stem cell research guidelines, several states such as California, Massachusetts, and New York have incorporated additional state-specific stem cell research regulations. Many countries, such as the United Kingdom, Canada, South Korea, and Singapore, have their own national stem cell research regulations. I do not wish in this chapter to cover all the regulations around the world. Instead I use the NAS and ISSCR guidelines as focal points to concentrate our attention on broader themes relating to practical research ethics.

of human research subjects.[2] The second major outcome of the act was the establishment of the National Commission for the Protection of Human Subjects of Biomedical and Behavioral Research, a group of scholars, physicians, and lawyers assembled to identify basic ethical principles underlying all human subjects research. The National Commission issued its report in 1979, widely referred to today as the Belmont Report. In this report the authors highlighted the importance of respect for persons, beneficence, and justice – as discussed in Chapter 3. The Belmont Report recommended that each of these basic moral principles could be practically applied to the conduct of research through the institutional regulatory requirements of informed consent, risk-benefit assessment, and fair subject selection.

These two main effects of the National Research Act – the requirement for IRB review and the conclusions of the Belmont Report – eventually came together in the form of the U.S. Federal Policy for the Protection of Human Subjects (45 CFR 46) issued by the Department of Health and Human Services and overseen by the Office of Human Research Protections. These federal regulations now constitute the American national standard for human subjects research.[3] This policy is usually referred to as the Common Rule, and it requires human subjects research to be reviewed by an IRB. An IRB is charged with upholding the Belmont Report principles by reviewing aspects of a proposed study relating to informed consent, risk-benefit ratio assessment, and fair subject selection.

Notably, the Common Rule applies only to human subjects research that is federally related in one way or another. That is, a proposed study is subject to the Common Rule only if one of these three conditions holds: (1) the study is either conducted or funded by the federal government; (2) the study is conducted at an institution such as a university or research hospital that has pledged conformity with the Common Rule for all its research; or (3) the study falls within the jurisdiction of the FDA because it involves an investigational new drug, device, or more

[2] Other countries have committees similar to this referred to as Ethical Review Boards.
[3] At the time of this writing, however, the U.S. Department of Health and Human Services and the Office of Science and Technology Policy have proposed a series of changes to the rules governing human subjects oversight (Berg and Deming 2011). Proposed revisions include improving data security and adverse event reporting; broadening informed consent to allow for more open-ended uses of stored biological specimens; and extending federal regulations to all U.S. research regardless of funding source. The impact of these proposed changes on stem cell research is unknown at this point because the nature and scope of the relevant changes are still under deliberation.

than minimally manipulated biologic. Exceptions to the Common Rule requirement are if (1) the study is neither conducted nor funded by the federal government; (2) it is not conducted at an institution that has contractually committed itself to apply the Common Rule; and (3) the study does not come within the jurisdiction of the FDA.

It is important to recognize that there are many types of stem cell research that, if neither related to federal funding nor subject to FDA regulation of complex biologics, would fall outside the scope of the Common Rule (Coleman et al. 2005). Such research may occur, for example, in IVF clinics and some private physicians' offices. This does not necessarily mean, however, that *no* research regulatory standard would pertain in such situations, because many states have passed their own laws similar to the Common Rule for any research that is conducted within their borders. For example, Louisiana prohibits the use of any remaining fertility clinic embryos for research, while California requires, through its Health and Safety Code, that all research involving the derivation and use of hES cells from any source (including SCNT) must be IRB reviewed. Nevertheless, in states without local laws approximating the Common Rule, there remains the concern that some clinicians conducting nonfederally related research may find loopholes for circumventing IRB review.

Another aspect of the Common Rule relevant for stem cell research ethics is its working definition of *human subjects research*. According to the Common Rule, human subjects research involves "a systematic investigation … designed to develop or contribute to generalizable knowledge and which uses living humans or identifiable information about living humans" (Rivera 2008). Clearly, this means that the requirements of IRB review and informed consent pertain to all stem cell research in which study leaders must interact with living human materials donors for the procurement of embryos, somatic cells, and other starting materials for stem cell derivation. But, importantly, the Common Rule also applies to *in vitro* stem cell research using human tissue samples or cells that are collected with identifiable private information. Information is considered identifiable if "the identity of the subject is or may readily be ascertained by the investigator or associated with the information" (45 CFR 46.102(f)(2)).

Human biological materials used in research can be grouped into one of four categories: (1) *anonymous samples*, which are provided to researchers from specimens initially collected without any individually identifying information; (2) *anonymized samples*, which are provided to researchers after individually indentifying information has been permanently removed by the storage facility; (3) *coded samples*, which are provided to researchers after individually identifying information has been replaced with a code by the storage facility, which retains the key to the code; and (4) *identified samples*, which are sent to researchers with individually identifying information.

Generally, the Common Rule applies to research involving human biological samples that can be linked to specific individuals either directly or indirectly through coding systems (categories 3 and 4). The only time research involving coded samples (category 3) would not be considered human subjects research is if (1) the key to decipher the code is destroyed before the research begins; (2) the investigators and the holder of the code enter into an mutual agreement not to release the decoding key to the investigators under any circumstances, or until the individuals are deceased; or (3) there are IRB-approved written policies for a tissue repository that prohibit the release of the decoding key to investigators under any circumstances or until the individuals are deceased (Office of Human Research Protections 2008).[4] Notice that, in regard to research with human biological materials, current federal requirements are limited mainly to the management of "informational risks." Informational risks are defined as the potential inappropriate disclosure or use of information that could be harmful to study subjects, such as the disclosure of private health information.

Each of the IRB-centered regulatory areas listed previously are important – informed consent, risk-benefit assessment, fair subject selection, and the management of informational risks. However, none of these areas, either alone or in combination, fully addresses all the ethical issues pertaining to stem cell research. As we saw in Chapter 2, a very large portion of stem cell research involves *in vitro* studies using coded biological specimens and established stem cell lines. The object of research in these tissue culture studies is not the human subject him- or herself but rather the plasticity potential of radically manipulated cells. Historically, research regulation in the United States arose as a response to the egregious exploitation of human subjects for medical research and observational studies of untreated diseases. But it was around this same time that, in what was practically a parallel biomedical universe, tissue culture

---

[4] Office of Human Research Protections, 2008. *Guidance on Research Involving Coded Private Information or Biological Specimens.* http://www.hhs.gov/ohrp/policy/cdebiol.html (accessed January 8, 2012).

research really began to come into its own. The nearly cotemporaneous development of human subjects regulations, on the one hand, and stem cell–relevant tissue culture research, on the other, proceeded along dual historical pathways; pathways that did not intersect until much later at the crossroads of having to manage the informational risks facing human biomaterials donors.

It is important to realize, however, that the range of ethical issues in basic stem cell research goes beyond concerns about informational risk. As I discuss in the following section, institutional research oversight is just now getting extended beyond traditional human subjects protections to include other policies governing basic stem cell research performed, not in human subjects, but in culture dishes and in animal systems.

## Toward Stem Cell–Specific Policies

The origins of current stem cell–specific guidelines follow a tradition of scientists and other academics coming together to devise ethical standards for a research field in light of new advances.[5] One of the most widely known examples of such self-guidance occurred in 1975 when a group of biologists held a meeting with physicians and lawyers to draft voluntary guidelines for the use of recombinant DNA technologies (Berg et al. 1975). A key principle articulated during this meeting (commonly referred to as the Asilomar Conference) was the notion that biosafety standards for recombinant DNA research ought to be proportionate to the levels of risk involved. To this end, meeting participants classified various forms of recombinant DNA research into separate categories ranging from minimal, low, medium, and high risk to prohibited research. The consensus standards that came out of this meeting had a lasting effect on the regulation of genetic research in the United States. The Asilomar Conference principles, in combination with the near simultaneous formation of the Recombinant DNA Advisory Committee (the RAC) by the NIH, have helped direct the federal oversight of recombinant DNA research to this present day.

Another example of professional self-guidance comes from the U.K. Committee of Inquiry into Human Fertilisation and Embryology (commonly referred to as the Warnock Committee). In 1982, four years after the birth of the first IVF baby in England, Parliament commissioned a group of scientists, philosophers, theologians, and lawyers

---

[5] We see other examples of this within the profession of medicine in Chapter 8.

to draft recommendations for the responsible use of assisted reproductive technologies and the conduct of human embryo research (Warnock 1985).[6] Among the many important guidelines issued in the Warnock Report, two recommendations stand out as particularly relevant for our discussion of stem cell research guidelines.

First, the Warnock Committee recommended that a new statutory licensing authority be established to regulate embryo research and infertility services. This recommendation resulted in the 1990 Human Fertilisation and Embryology Act, which in turn authorized the creation of the Human Fertilisation and Embryology Authority (HFEA). Today, the HFEA licenses all IVF procedures in the United Kingdom and controls all embryo research, including the derivation of hES cells.

Second, the Warnock Committee recommended that no embryo research be conducted on human embryos in culture beyond fourteen days after fertilization. Prior to the first fourteen days of development, research can be conducted on human embryos created through the IVF process, whether they are created initially for reproductive purposes and no longer needed by the couple or whether they are created specifically for research use. The Warnock Committee justified its fourteen-day limit on grounds that, prior to the formation of the primitive streak, a human embryo *in vitro* is not yet a distinct individual but rather retains the biologic potential to fuse and divide into different cellular masses (Cohen 2007; Warnock 1985). The primitive streak is an elongated band of cells that forms along the axis of the fertilized human egg after approximately

---

[6]  Among the members of the Warnock Committee was the renowned Cambridge developmental biologist Anne McLaren. Dame Professor McLaren first developed in 1958 the technique of IVF in mice, a process she used to study the developmental effects of maternal stress on mouse offspring during pregnancy (McLaren, personal communication). The technical advance of being able to create and grow embryos outside the maternal body eventually led to its application in humans by Drs. Edwards and Steptoe in 1978. Dame Professor McLaren contributed enormously to the drafting of the Warnock Report and testified often in Parliament on issues relating to human assisted reproduction, science, and ethics.

Dame Professor McLaren also had a significant impact many years later on the formation of the ISSCR guidelines for basic stem cell research discussed later in this chapter section. She served on the ISSCR subcommittee on human biological materials procurement, which I chaired in 2006. Her scientific expertise and experience were extremely valuable for our deliberations on the ethical procurement of embryos, gametes, and somatic cells for stem cell research. She died suddenly in 2007, immediately after she helped the ISSCR Ethics and Public Policy Committee think through our approach to human/animal chimera research, an approach that eventually developed into the ISSCR advisory report on chimeras that I discuss in Chapter 5. Her knowledge and wisdom are greatly missed.

fourteen consecutive days of development. This band of cells is the most rudimentary precursor to the embryo's neural tube and nervous system. The Warnock Committee recommended that, prior to the appearance of the primitive streak, an embryo can be used for scientifically justified research that may involve its destruction in the process. Bedsides the enduring regulatory regime of the HFEA, which the Warnock Committee helped to initiate, the Warnock Committee has also had the lasting legacy of having the fourteen-day limit rule adopted later in stem cell research guidelines in the United States and around the world.

In view of the positive regulatory impacts that professionally led efforts like Asilomar and the Warnock Committee have had in the past for controversial science, it was soon recognized by scientists in the United States that a similar self-guiding effort ought to take place for hES cell research. Unlike some countries, such as the United Kingdom, Japan, and Canada, the United States still had no national stem cell oversight commission or centrally authorized committee (similar to the RAC) to guide and review stem cell research (Cohen 2007). In 2005, given the absence of harmonized ethical standards at the national level, the U.S. National Academy of Sciences (NAS) volunteered to produce a series of nonbinding guidelines for the ethical conduct of hES cell research (National Academy of Sciences 2005). Written by a cohort of prominent American scientists, legal specialists, and bioethicists, the NAS guidelines set forth ethical recommendations for all university, industry, and private-sector researchers who derive and/or use hES cell lines. Its major recommendations include voluntary institutional oversight of hES cell research in the form of Embryonic Stem Cell Research Oversight (ESCRO) committees, and enhanced IRB review of the procurement of human biological materials (eggs, sperm, embryos, or somatic cells) used to derive new hES cell lines.

The ESCRO committees today are comprised of scientific, legal, and bioethical experts, plus community representatives. Their purpose is several-fold. However, each of these functions should be understood as converging on the overarching aim of providing stem cell–specific expertise and review of aspects of hES cell research that may otherwise escape traditional regulatory mechanisms.

According to the NAS guidelines, ESCROs are meant to complement existing IRBs and Institutional Animal Care and Use Committees (IACUCs) in the oversight of hES cell research protocols directly involving human volunteers or laboratory animals. The ESCRO committees are supposed to coordinate the review of all stem cell research–based informed consent procedures with IRBs (although it is not specified exactly in what manner), particularly those aimed at procuring human biological materials to derive new hES cell lines. For studies in which hES cells are transferred into postnatal animals or gestating fetal animals, ESCROs are tasked with coordinating the review and approval of these studies with IACUCs, taking into special account the likely developmental integration of human cells into nonhuman animal tissues systems. (Again, the exact nature of this coordinated review is not specified in the NAS guidelines.)

Besides providing stem cell expertise for coordinated IRB and IACUC reviews, ESCRO committees are also responsible for overseeing *in vitro* hES cell research. *In vitro* research, by definition, does not directly involve experimental animals; thus, it falls outside the remit of an IACUC. Moreover, aside from informed consent requirements for human materials donors and the management of informational risks, IRBs have little else to do with overseeing *in vitro* hES cell research. Thus ESCRO committees are meant to provide oversight for *in vitro* stem cell research that would otherwise fall between the cracks of IRB and IACUC review.

To date, ESCRO committees have stepped in to help fill this research oversight gap for stem cell science. The NAS guidelines have become widely influential in the United States, with nearly every institution involved with hES cell research voluntarily subjecting itself to ESCRO committee review. In addition, all state granting agencies and many scientific journals now make it a condition for project funding or publication that researchers provide assurance of their having received ESCRO committee approval.

A year after the NAS guidelines, in late 2006, a similar set of guidelines for hES cell research was released by the ISSCR. The purpose of these guidelines was to articulate a set of ethical and professional standards for pluripotent stem cell research which, in the spirit of self-regulation, was directed toward the international scientific community that comprises the ISSCR (Daley et al. 2007). The ISSCR guidelines were drafted by a task force composed of scientists, ethicists, and legal experts representing fourteen different countries active in stem cell research (International Society for Stem Cell Research 2006). Like the NAS committee, the ISSCR task force had no political or legal authority, so it could only offer general professional guidelines for the conduct of human pluripotent stem cell research, not regulations. Regulations offer a set of standards for which one can either be in or out of compliance, and for which there exists an enforcement mechanism wielded by a recognized authority. Guidelines, in contrast, are a set of broad recommendations, expectations, and aspirational goals for right conduct, but are not enforceable in the way of regulations. What follows is a highlighted summary of the ISSCR guidelines, including their key differences with the NAS guidelines.

*Independent Oversight*

Like the NAS, the ISSCR recommends that a specialized SCRO process be implemented to complement existing institutional boards lacking such stem cell–specific review. Unlike the NAS, however, the ISSCR does not stipulate that institutions form and utilize ESCRO committees per se, but rather that they employ key elements of a single stem cell research oversight (SCRO) process that examines all research involving the derivation and use of pluripotent human stem cells.[7] In some countries, governmental bodies already exist to oversee this research, such as the HFEA. In light of such international variation, the ISSCR guidelines recommend simply that there ought to be a single stem cell research review process at the institutional, regional, or national level (whichever is pertinent to the country in question) in order to provide independent and specialized oversight while avoiding redundancy. Regardless of the level at which the SCRO process occurs, individuals who carry out the SCRO function should include (1) scientists and/or physicians with relevant expertise in stem cell biology, assisted reproduction, developmental biology, and clinical medicine; (2) ethicists with expertise in research ethics; (3) legal experts familiar with local laws governing research; and (4) community members unaffiliated with the research under review or the researchers' institution.

The key elements to be considered under SCRO review are the scientific rationale and merit of the research proposal, the relevant expertise of the investigators, and the ethical permissibility of the research. With respect to this last element – ethical permissibility – the ISSCR guidelines outline specific categories of research that the SCRO review process is meant to identify and assess.

---

[7] Notice that the ISSCR guidelines employ the SCRO acronym rather than the ESCRO acronym. The ISSCR guidelines task force dropped the term *embryonic* from the name of the oversight process to indicate that the SCRO function could cover pluripotent stem cells that may not be embryonic in origin, thus presaging the arrival of human iPS cells a few years later.

*Permissible and Impermissible Research*

The ISSCR guidelines outline the varieties of research that, in principle, would be permissible after SCRO review. The guidelines also identify certain forms of research that would be prohibited in all circumstances. From a SCRO point of view, all basic research using human pluripotent stem cells can be sorted into one of these three categories.

Category 1 denotes research that would be permissible after an expedited administrative review, such as *in vitro* studies using an established human pluripotent stem cell line. Full SCRO committee review is not necessary for Category 1 research; rather, an expedited SCRO review is meant to focus mainly on assurances that the established human pluripotent stem cell line to be studied *in vitro* was derived in a manner consistent with any applicable IRB and legal requirements and with the donor informed consent procedures of the ISSCR guidelines (see my discussion of these consent procedures in the following text).

Category 2 research is any research that is subject to full SCRO review. Unlike Category 1, this type of research requires greater levels of scientific justification and a careful consideration of its social and ethical aspects. Category 2 research involves any of the following activities: (1) the derivation of new human pluripotent stem cell lines by any means, (2) research in which the identity of human materials donors is readily ascertainable to the investigator, (3) human stem cell–based chimera research, or (4) clinical research in which human pluripotent stem cells or their direct derivatives are transplanted into human subjects. The derivation of new human pluripotent stem cell lines triggers the need for SCRO committees to coordinate with an IRB in order to ensure that stem cell–specific information is appropriately introduced into the donor consent process. The use of identifiable human materials similarly triggers the need for a SCRO assurance that relevant IRB requirements are met that relate to human tissues research (see the preceding discussion concerning IRB oversight of biological samples research). Human stem cell–based chimera research – particularly experiments that are likely to produce extensive chimerism of the nonhuman animal brain and/or gonads – warrants full SCRO review of the developmental possibilities, ethical implications, and other factors not typically deliberated upon by animal use (IACUC) review committees. (I focus further on this aspect of SCRO review in Chapter 5.) Finally, the ISSCR guidelines call upon SCRO committees to use their stem cell–specific expertise to review clinical research in which pluripotent stem cells or their direct derivatives are introduced into human subjects.

Importantly, this last requirement has been effectively dropped from the Category 2 designation upon the 2008 release of the ISSCR *Guidelines for the Clinical Translation of Stem Cells.* The ISSCR clinical translation guidelines map out in greater detail the ethical and professional benchmarks for stem cell–based interventional human subjects research, and they limit the role of the SCRO process in this area. I discuss these standards and other important issues in Chapters 7 and 8.

In summary, Category 2 research practically boils down to the review of two main areas: proposed derivations of new pluripotent stem cell lines and human/nonhuman chimera research in which there is a possibility of human cells integrating into the CNSs and/or the germ lines of laboratory animals.[8] Research using human stem cells with readily identifiable information is not so much a focus of SCRO review today, because IRBs normally oversee and approve such research, with little value added to this process by SCRO committees. In the future, however, with the development of "clinical grade" stem cells and their derivatives (see Chapter 2), there may come a need for SCRO review of any proposals for long-term donor tracking to ensure the quality and genetic safety of the stem cell products derived from their donated biological materials.

Category 3 denotes research that should not be pursued at this time. The ISSCR identifies three forms of prohibited research. First, following the fourteen-day limit articulated by the Warnock Committee, the ISSCR guidelines explicitly prohibit the *in vitro* culture of a human embryo beyond fourteen consecutive days of development or the formation of the primitive embryonic streak. Unlike the NAS guidelines, which prohibit the mixing of cells of any nature with the prestreak human embryo, the ISSCR guidelines allow for such experiments, but only if they have a sound scientific rationale and follow the fourteen-day limit. Second, the ISSCR guidelines prohibit experiments in which any products of research involving human pluripotent stem cells are implanted into a human or nonhuman primate uterus. And third, research may not be conducted in which animal chimeras incorporating human cells with the potential to form gametes are bred to one another. These last two restrictions are in place to avoid any unpredictable and ethically

---

[8] Unlike the NAS guidelines, which require full SCRO review of all chimera research, the ISSCR guidelines exempt human stem cell teratoma assays in immune-deficient mice from full committee review (Lensch et al. 2007). These assays are considered routine practice for characterizing the quality of human pluripotent stem cells (see Chapter 2); thus, the ISSCR task force decided to subsume these tests under Category 1 research.

concerning research outcomes in which morally ambiguous forms of biological life are artificially generated and birthed into existence. (I address the philosophical and ethical limits of these concerns in Chapter 5.)

*Informed Consent*

The ISSCR guidelines recognize the importance of the public's participation in human pluripotent stem cell research. Most commonly, public participation consists of the donation and provision of necessary starting materials for the derivation of new stem cell lines (preimplantation embryos, gametes, and somatic cells). To ensure that the procurement of these materials is conducted in a manner consistent with current ethical standards for informed consent, and to encourage the implementation of additional stem cell–specific considerations during the consent process, the ISSCR guidelines recommend the following.

First, consent for the donation of biological materials should be obtained very close to the proposed time in which the materials are to be transferred to the research team. This call for "contemporaneous consent" includes the need to obtain consent from any third-party gamete donors involved in the creation of fertility clinic embryos that may later be used for research. Third-party gamete donors who provide sperm or eggs for assisted reproductive purposes may object to their inadvertent participation in supporting hES cell research, and for this reason they need to be recontacted and consented specifically for their possible complicit involvement in stem cell research.[9]

The only exception to this contemporaneous consent recommendation is in cases in which researchers obtain somatic cells from a tissue bank to derive new stem cell lines. However, this exception only applies if the tissue bank supplying the somatic cells indicates on its own donor consent forms the possibility that their banked tissues may be used to

---

[9] I am told by many researchers, however, that this recommendation to obtain informed consent from third-party gamete donors prior to embryo procurement for stem cell research is nearly impossible to fulfill. Most third-party gamete donors are anonymous, and it is very difficult to track down these individuals to obtain their consent in a timely manner to procure any embryos resulting from their contributed gametes. Due to this practical difficulty, many stem cell researchers have decided only to procure remaining embryos from couples who did not use third-party gamete donors. Unfortunately, in many of these circumstances either the man or the woman has fertility problems (hence their need to use IVF technology), and researchers are not sure what effect these problems may have on the quality of the embryonic stem cells derived from their leftover and often subclinical embryos.

create new pluripotent stem cell lines and if researchers only use tissue samples whose donors have clearly consented to this possible use.[10]

Other highlights from the ISSCR guidelines include factors that aim to bolster the informed consent dialogue for human materials donors. To this end, representatives of the research team must review several important discussion points with potential research donors at the time of the informed consent interview. For example, embryo donors specifically should be told that their donated IVF embryos will be destroyed during the process of hES cell derivation. Also, donors for all types of materials must be informed that the resulting stem cell lines will be shared with researchers at different institutions for other ethically reviewed research purposes, the scientific aims of which are largely unknown at this time. Donors should also be told whether there are any plans for researchers to share with them commercial royalties resulting from later applications of the derived stem cells. And all donors must be made aware of their alternatives to donating human materials for research. Potential donors must know that, whatever decision they make, the quality of their own medical care will not be affected.[11]

Although the NAS guidelines promulgate a very similar set of informed consent standards, the ISSCR guidelines depart by adding further recommendations for ways regulators and researchers can improve the practice of informed consent. Informed consent should be viewed as an ongoing process of dialogue with potential research donors, not simply a one-time event resulting in the signing of a contractual document. To improve the quality of this interactive dialogue, the ISSCR guidelines recommend that, whenever possible, the person conducting the informed consent interview should have no vested interest in the research protocol. This is to help minimize the possibility of biasing the potential donor's understanding of the risks and benefits of research participation. Also, counseling services should be made available upon request to any human materials donor prior to procurement. And all procurement procedures should be reviewed periodically and improved

---

[10] To my knowledge, I am not aware of any tissue banks that have revised their consent forms in this recommended manner.

[11] There are too many other details for me to cover adequately in this section. Readers should refer to the *ISSCR Guidelines for the Conduct of hESC Research*, especially section 11. Also readers should consult the informed consent form templates I developed for the ISSCR for embryo, egg, and somatic cell donation, available at http://www.isscr.org/AM/Template.cfm?Section=GuidelinesforhESCResearch&Template=/CM/ContentDisplay.cfm&ContentID=2230 (accessed December 1, 2011).

in light of new sociological studies or experiences pertaining to donors' understanding of their participation in stem cell research.

*Egg-Provider Compensation*

The ISSCR and the NAS offer differing guidelines on the controversial issue of egg-provider payments. According to the NAS, women who undergo hormonal induction to provide eggs directly for SCNT research may only receive reimbursements for their out-of-pocket expenses. Compensation – that is, payment for their time, effort, and inconvenience – is prohibited. The ISSCR guidelines, by contrast, recommend more generally that financial considerations of any kind must not constitute an undue inducement, and that at no time should payments be given for the number and quality of the research eggs. Independent ethical review is also strongly recommended to provide assurance of these requirements (Daley et al. 2007). In this way, the ISSCR guidelines leave open the possibility for ethics review committees to permit egg-provider compensation after reviewing a study team's proposed payment levels and recruitment practices (Hyun 2006b; 2011b).[12] Although some critics may believe that the ISSCR departs from usual practice in this regard, the fact is that this aspect of the ISSCR guidelines better accords with ethical practices in other areas of biomedical science, in which people who provide human biological research materials through invasive surgical procedures are proportionately compensated for their time, effort, and inconvenience (Crockin 2010).

*Research Sharing*

Like the NAS, the ISSCR recommends that researchers ought to make their stem cell lines readily accessible to other investigators in the

---

[12] In 2009 the Empire State Stem Cell Board in New York State embodied the ISSCR guidelines by permitting state funds to be used for egg-provider compensation in stem cell research after appropriate ethics committee approval (Roxland 2012).

In contrast, Massachusetts legally prohibits researchers from compensating egg providers in that state. Stem cell scientists at Harvard tried for years to recruit altruistic egg donors in compliance with state law and the NAS guidelines (Kevin Eggan, personal communication). However, this lengthy "social experiment" turned out to be a flat out failure, with only one altruistic egg donor ever being recruited (Egli et al. 2011). These sustained efforts confirmed what many of us had suspected all along – that women typically are not willing to endure hormonal induction for research simply in exchange for validated parking tickets, reimbursed meals, and a pat on the back (Klitzman and Sauer 2009). What outside observers should learn from this experience is that we do not live in a world in which our policy choice is between altruistic egg donation, on the one hand, and compensation, on the other. In the actual world, our true alternatives are fair compensation or a dearth of eggs for research.

biomedical research community. Thus the ISSCR guidelines include a call for harmonized international standards for derivation, banking, storage, and distribution of research materials. However, unlike the NAS, the ISSCR recommends further that stem cell lines should be internationally distributed and shared free of charge, aside from the necessary costs of shipping and handling. This last provision is justified by the aspirational ideal that human stem cell research ought to benefit society and the humanitarian advancement of science as much as possible. Arguably, this lofty goal may be best promoted when research materials are widely shared at low cost to the research community.

## New Directions, New Questions

Having covered most of the major elements of the ISSCR and NAS guidelines, it is important to acknowledge that the SCRO mechanism for research oversight is still evolving. Many SCRO committees have experienced new questions arising from the fact that human pluripotent stem cell research has advanced considerably in the past few years.

### Stem Cell Research Oversight Authority and Reach

One issue that demands careful consideration is whether and to what extent iPS cell research ought to be overseen by SCRO committees. It is interesting to note that the ISSCR and NAS guidelines were developed prior to the advent of iPS cell technology. Now that new human pluripotent stem cell lines can be derived without the use of embryos, there is some controversy among SCRO committees as to whether pluripotent *nonembryonic* stem cell research needs to meet SCRO approval. Some would assert that ESCRO and SCRO committees were first devised in response to the ethical and social sensitivities surrounding the use of human embryos in stem cell research. Critics may argue further that if iPS cell research had developed first, before hES cell research, we would not be questioning today whether iPS cells research should fall under SCRO review. It should be admitted that this counterfactual may defy the very likelihood of iPS cell research, given the latter's scientific debt to our knowledge about hES cells (see Chapter 2). Nevertheless, the main point of this critique seems to be that it is the embryonic source of stem cells that gives SCRO committees their *raison d'être*. Others may argue in response that the pluripotent properties of iPS cells are sufficient to justify their need to be overseen by SCRO committees. If iPS cells have the same potentially controversial research applications as hES cells, then it is proper to require SCRO oversight for iPS and hES cells.

This latter view is, in my opinion, the correct one. As I suggested in Chapter 2, stem cells should be defined, not by their source, but by their potential, that is, by the range of their ability to be manipulated into other cell types. Accepting this claim, however, could lead us down a slippery path of regulatory indeterminacy. Others may sense that we are already on this slippery path. For instance, there is growing confusion among many SCRO committees about the point at which they need to stop overseeing research on mature cells that have been differentiated many cell types away from their original pluripotent stem cells. How far down the stem cell differentiation chain does the authority of SCRO committees extend? Does it stop when researchers use multipotent stem cells derived from pluripotent cells? Does it stop when researchers use pluripotent stem cell–derived multipotent cells to create, for example, red blood cell progenitors? Does it stop when researchers propose to use mature blood cells derived from these progenitor cells? And so on.

Suppose one draws the SCRO review line somewhere around the pluripotent stem cell–derived multipotent cell stage. Then other vexing questions begin to creep in. For example, if SCRO committees review *in vitro* and animal research involving human neural stem cells derived from either hES or iPS cells, then what about research involving neural stem cells harvested from human brains post mortem? Because SCRO committee review is limited only to research involving pluripotent stem cells and their direct derivatives, there would be no extension of SCRO authority over multipotent stem cell research utilizing cells harvested from fully formed organ systems. But if the research uses and ethical issues surrounding neural stem cells are largely the same, regardless of whether they were derived from pluripotent stem cells or harvested from donated human brains, then treating the two sets of neural stem cells differently at the institutional review level seems arbitrary. How would one resolve this difficulty without overextending the authority of the SCRO committee?

Aside from these difficult SCRO issues, there are other practical questions swirling around the ethics of human materials donation. These practical ethical questions resist any quick solutions, for they are ultimately tied to deep philosophical uncertainties about the moral reach of deontological and consequentialist reasons and the limits they can place on one another (see Chapter 1). I have space here only to identify these new problems and offer some tentative comments about the directions I think these emerging issues might take.

*Donor Withdrawal and Control*

One challenging issue concerns the nature and limits of what it means for human materials donors to participate in stem cell research.[13] Does research participation entitle a donor to withdraw later – perhaps very much later – a resulting pluripotent stem cell line from all research uses?[14] Similarly, does research participation mean that an original donor can direct what kind of research can and cannot be performed using a resulting stem cell line?[15] At what stage of the research regulation process should this issue be managed, by scientists during the study design phase of the research, by the IRB, or by the SCRO committee? Let us begin by addressing the first question.

Traditionally, research ethics allows research participants the right to withdraw themselves from a scientific project at any time for any reason. But normally this right presumes that human subjects research involves ongoing scientific activities performed on the participant's *body* such that research withdrawal is intimately connected to a person's right to bodily integrity and sovereignty (personal autonomy). Typically in these cases, when a human research subject decides to withdraw from a study, the normal course of action is rather straightforward – researchers must stop the experimental intervention on that person and remove him or her from the research project. In most human subjects research, such as clinical trials, the issue of subject withdrawal and the conditions necessitating its implementation are usually addressed together by the research

[13] This is the topic of an advisory report being drafted by the ISSCR Ethics and Public Policy Committee. The viewpoints expressed are my own and do not necessarily reflect the opinions of the committee.

[14] Currently, most informed consent forms for human materials donation specify that donors can withdraw their embryos, somatic cells, or unfertilized eggs from research up until these materials are transferred to the research team and prepared for stem cell derivation. The preceding question, however, concerns whether original donors can withdraw a resulting stem cell line from research after derivation has taken place. Obviously if one answers "yes" to this question, one would have to recommend dropping the current wording of informed consent forms that limit donor withdrawal to the time at which the donated human materials are transferred to the research team.

[15] The NAS and ISSCR guidelines allow for this possibility, but to my knowledge this is not a practice that has been actualized by any research team, at least not on purpose. One of Doug Melton's hES cell lines at Harvard was obtained from an informed consent procedure that explained to potential embryo donors that the resulting stem cell lines would be used for research on endoderm development (Chad Cowan, personal communication). The NIH stem cell registry working group has interpreted this wording to mean that this particular hES cell line can *only* be used for endoderm research (Terry Magnuson, personal communication).

team during the design of their study and by the IRB (see Chapter 7). Although there will always be safety and health monitoring issues and the like to be concerned with, responsible research withdrawal typically does not raise the sort of questions posed by stem cell research regarding what it means *philosophically* for original donors to be involved as "participants" in ongoing tissue culture studies.

Some may point out that similar questions have been asked about what it means for persons to participate in genetic studies involving their private genetic information. Some may argue that participants in genetic studies have a moral right to withdraw their genetic samples from research at any point, even if these samples have been coded to protect their privacy. This position seems to be based on the belief that individuals have an autonomy interest in controlling the uses of their own genetic information. In the same way that an individual can autonomously opt out of research conducted on his or her body at any point, so too can an individual autonomously opt out of allowing researchers to conduct studies on his or her genetic samples. A person's right to autonomy governs, so the argument goes, decisions over the research uses of one's own body as well as the research uses of one's DNA, regardless of whether the DNA samples have been removed long ago from one's physical self.

Although the preceding views can be controversial, I generally tend to agree with this line of reasoning as it applies to genetic research. However, my chief concern is that there may be key differences between genetic research and pluripotent stem cell research that would make an analogous conclusion harder to draw for the latter.

First, there is the complicating fact that pluripotent stem cell lines may have differing degrees of genetic similarity to their original donors depending on how these lines were derived and whether they were genetically altered for research purposes. The presence of either of these two variables would weaken attempts to extend the genetic studies analogy to some types of stem cell research original donors. Why?

Our ability to extend the genetic research analogy to stem cell original donors relies on a simple but important presupposition – namely, that the strength of a donor's rightful claim to withdraw a biological sample from research depends directly on whether that person's genetic information is actually contained in that sample. We assume that, in the case of genetic research, such a corresponding link must exist between the genetic sample and the genetic donor. Thus a donor has a strong right to exclude the use of a genetic research sample only if that sample is a genetic match to him or her. The reason why this (often unstated) dependency relation is important is because the rights claim at issue here is a type of autonomy right.[16] If this general approach to understanding research sample withdrawal is correct, then the following outcomes would result across the range of various pluripotent stem cell derivation techniques.

Embryo donors for stem cell research would have a much-reduced claim to autonomously withdraw any hES cell lines derived from their donated embryos. Unlike genetic donors, whose biological samples are 100 percent genetically matched to them, no embryo donor can claim to have more than a 50 percent match to any derived hES cell line. The situation gets more complicated once we recognize that embryo donation can involve multiple deciding parties, any one of whom may veto the use of an embryo for stem cell research according to current NAS and ISSCR guidelines: the couple for whom the IVF embryo was created and who has dispositional authority over it and any third-party gamete donors whose genetic contribution helped create the embryo. If it is true that the strength of any stem cell withdrawal rights exists in proportion to the degree of personal genetic information contained in the research sample (this is a debatable point, I know), then this logic would militate against recognizing all stem cell withdrawal rights as being fully comparable to the withdrawal rights of donors in genetic research.

Furthermore, this approach would leave some original donors with no withdrawal rights at all over stem cell lines based on a shared-genetics rationale. Most notably, this limitation would involve IVF treatment couples who use third-party gamete donors for both their sperm and eggs and SCNT egg providers who contribute no personal genetic information to the resulting stem cell line aside from their mitochondrial DNA.[17]

---

[16] Parents of pediatric patients have the right to withdraw their child's genetic sample from research without their child's personal authorization to do so. But this practice can be justified on the grounds of parental autonomy rights that protect the authority of parental decisions concerning a child's best interests. Parental decision-making authority remains in place as long as parents are not negligent and the child lacks the ability to exercise his or her autonomy. So an autonomy defense of parental rights to withdraw pediatric genetic samples could be reasonably offered here in a roundabout manner. Furthermore, parents could also claim a shared veto right to exclude their child's genetic samples from research, much in the way that gamete donors can share veto rights in the embryo donation scenario for stem cell research discussed in the following paragraph.

[17] However it is worth noting that, in the only published human SCNT study thus far (Noggle et al. 2011), researchers had to leave the egg providers' maternal DNA in their unfertilized eggs prior to somatic cell nuclear transfer. Thus the resulting SCNT stem cell lines from this study contained the genetics of the egg provider and the genetics of the somatic cell provider. See my discussion of this research protocol in Chapter 2, note 14.

However, for somatic cell donors in iPS cell and SCNT studies, each derived stem cell line would be a genetic match to each somatic cell donor. Thus the rationale for allowing somatic cell donors to withdraw stem cell lines aligns with the rationale for allowing genetic donors to withdraw their samples from genetic research, assuming that the resulting iPS cell or SCNT stem cell line has not been genetically altered for research purposes.

There are probably other types of arguments aside from the genetic link rationale I outlined in the preceding text that could support original donors' rights to withdraw stem cell lines. But whatever these other reasons specifically might be, I believe they all could be reduced to some variant of an individual's right to exercise personal autonomy.[18] If this assertion is correct, then all ethical arguments supporting an original donor's right to withdraw a stem cell line would ultimately have to address the following question. Does a donor's right to personal autonomy include dispositional rights of withdrawal and control over biological samples that have been radically transformed in the process of pluripotent stem cell derivation and cultivation?

In order for any autonomy-based argument to support either research withdrawal or donor control over future uses, there must exist a strong metaphysical connection between the individual and the research sample in question. In the case of genetic research, the connection between these two is rather tight. But in the case of pluripotent stem cell research (much of which involves quite radical biological transformations, as we saw in Chapter 2), the exact nature of the metaphysical connection between donor and research sample gets thrown into doubt. Recall that one of the chief scientific benefits of tissue culture research is that scientists can take a one-time biological donation and serially culture the sample to produce several future generations of research material without ever having to go back to the original donor. In this way, tissues in culture begin to take on a life of their own quite apart from the original donor. In the case of pluripotent stem cell research, cells in culture can be manipulated very far to a point where they are no longer the same type of cells or tissue as the original sample. For example, an iPS cell

---

[18] A purely consequentialist mode of defending a donor's "right" to withdraw research materials (genes and stem cells) is inadequate because it does not protect the donor's right to do so as a right in and of itself but as just one consideration among many in the overall weighing of benefits and burdens, and it would fall short of justifying one's refusal in the face of scientifically and socially valuable research. This latter point is a version of the aggregate effect I discuss in Chapter 7.

line can undergo more than forty-five doublings of cells, and most of these clonal iPS cells can be differentiated into a wide array of cell types. Does the somatic cell donor have reach-through rights over all these resulting cells?

Some people may argue that having the same nuclear genetic profile to a stem cell line is sufficient to justify a somatic cell donor's reach-through rights to withdraw or control an SCNT or iPS cell line. But I think this reasoning may be too hasty. What about the ongoing laboratory interventions and developmental pathway manipulations that are necessary for pluripotent stem cells to be maintained in culture? Without these constant interventions and manipulations, pluripotent stem cells would cease to exist physically as an object of study. Should these necessary and coordinated efforts carry any weight in one's determination of whether somatic cell donors have an exclusive right to withdraw stem cell lines? I believe they do, for the presence of these dynamic influences makes stem cell research disanalogous to plain genetic research per se. Some philosophers may go so far as to defend stem cell researchers by invoking a vaguely Lockean argument according to which researchers have accrued considerable private property interests in their derived stem cell lines because they have already "mixed their labor" with these cultured cells to a very high degree.

This is a complicated issue. Somatic cell donors and stem cell researchers might each reasonably claim to have property rights over the derived stem cell lines. Deciding who has the stronger claim will depend on which factor one judges to be determinative, having a genetic link to the stem cells or having established a record of creative technical labor to bring these cells into being. This issue is further complicated by the likelihood that clinical translational researchers may need to maintain long-term donor tracking for health information that might be relevant for the safe clinical use of any resulting stem cell lines and their derivatives. If somatic cell donors are to be burdened with this request as a condition of their participation in stem cell research, then it would seem difficult to justify not granting these donors some degree of control over future research use. The trick is to know how to balance all of these considerations into a single coherent and justifiable policy.

Some observers may point out that all of this could be sorted out through the informed consent process. I believe there is some truth to this. I have had enough practical experience helping researchers draft informed consent procedures to know how some of the difficulties outlined in the preceding text could be avoided in practice. For example, one approach would be to encourage researchers to disclose their intention of only enrolling donors who agree to waive their right to withdraw any derived stem cell lines from research use, as well as their right to control their future research uses (assuming such rights exist). The wording of the consent form could be expressed as follows: "Although some research teams may allow original donors to withdraw derived stem cell lines from research use at any point in the future, or to control their future research uses, our research team acknowledges that we cannot guarantee either of these possibilities for our donors. If you are uncomfortable with our position on this matter, you should not agree to participate as a human materials donor for our project."

Wording such as this should not be interpreted as a sneaky attempt by researchers to shrug off important moral rights of the donor. In many cases, stem cell researchers cannot control how researchers at other institutions will ultimately use the derived stem cells or their direct derivatives; neither can they force other researchers to stop using the derived cells, especially if other researchers have dramatically transformed these cells using methods they have patented in their own laboratories. I believe these realities present significant practical limitations on what a research team can promise to an original donor during the consent process. It may be misleading to suggest to a potential donor that he or she can actually retain autonomous control over a resulting stem cell line once it has been shared with others. Making such a promise to donors may, at best, be an empty gesture. At worst, obtaining informed consent from a donor on the basis of such a shaky promise may be morally pernicious, for it could undermine the authenticity of the informed consent process.[19] Some critics may argue that these practical limitations can be overcome. Some might claim that a research team can easily provide room for their original donors' preferences in the material transfer agreements (MTAs) that accompany each stem cell line distributed to other researchers. However, those on the other side of the issue may object that it would be too burdensome to try to monitor and enforce every single one of these donor preferences stipulated in the language of the MTA. Others may raise the more philosophical argument that

---

[19] A very similar argument has been made by bioethicists in the context of clinical ethics (Stein et al. 1996). Some have maintained that an advance offer of cardiopulmonary resuscitation (CPR), in futile cases in which CPR is not going to succeed, effectively amounts to presenting patients and their families with a false alternative. Allowing patient medical decision making to proceed on the basis of a false alternative undermines patient autonomy.

allowing donor restrictions on the specific uses of derived stem cell lines runs counter to the spirit of "open science" and open research use that is sanctioned within the ISSCR guidelines. The ability for scientists to pursue ethically reviewed research that they, not the original donors, deem to be important is crucial for the advancement of socially beneficial scientific research. This last brand of argument essentially pits the value of broad social benefit (beneficence) against the autonomy rights of original donors to control stem cell lines (assuming such autonomy rights exist). Whether the practical limitations of honoring donor preferences can be resolved through carefully worded MTAs does nothing to address this deeper philosophical controversy.

There are limitations to what informed consent documents and MTAs can resolve through their structure and wording. The careful wording of these documents does not disarm underlying philosophical questions about whether the conditions spelled out therein are ethically justified. It is possible for people to sign unfair informed consent forms and MTAs. Signing these documents does not automatically render unfair contracts fair. In order to know how to separate fair contracts from unfair contracts, we first have to wrestle with underlying ethical questions concerning the range of an original donor's autonomy rights over radically manipulated stem cell lines and their derivatives, and the ethical justifications supporting researchers' unrestricted use of these lines. The practical wording of documents cannot resolve these philosophical questions, even if ethical review committees allow these documents to be used for stem cell research.

### Donor Royalties

Another, perhaps more controversial, ethical issue involves the question of whether somatic cell donors for iPS cell and SCNT research deserve a share of any royalties resulting from the commercial applications of the resulting stem cell lines. Some commentators may argue that they do – that somatic cell donors are "co-producers in the generation of knowledge" and as such deserve some share of the profits (Solbakk 2011).[20] Disease-specific pluripotent stem cell lines are a hot commodity in the commercial world of drug screening and pharmaceutical drug

[20] Jan Helge Solbakk directs this claim toward egg providers for SCNT studies, but I think his position applies equally well, perhaps even better, to somatic cell donors. Readers should be aware that the ISSCR guidelines allow the potential for original donors to receive commercial royalties (see section 11.3a, viii). The NAS guidelines, however, discourage this possibility (see Recommendation 18h).

development (as discussed in Chapter 2). This raises a very provocative question. If every participant is getting paid in the process, from the suppliers providing reagents and cell culture systems, to principal investigators, staff, and postdoctoral students, to universities and biotechnology and drug companies, then why not also the somatic cell donors who initially provided the starting biological materials? After all, the somatic cell donor's biological specimen is arguably the most important component of the iPS cell derivation process used to produce disease-specific pluripotent stem cells.

Here again we run into the question of whether the informed consent contract can help resolve this ethical issue. My view is that it cannot. Even if the consent form is worded in a way that informs the donor not to expect any future commercial benefits arising from his or her somatic cell donation, still we may ask whether this financial exclusion of the donor is fair. By contrast, IRBs and SCRO committees clearly seem to have no problem with including such a stipulation. Every informed consent form I am aware of used in stem cell derivation protocols explicitly discloses the researchers' intent not to share with the donor any royalties resulting from future commercial uses. It is interesting to note, however, that there exist no practical barriers to providing somatic cell donors a share of future stem cell royalties. But time and time again researchers and regulators have made a choice not to do so. Why?

It appears that the current ethical default policy of not allowing donor royalties is grounded in a couple of consequentialist concerns. First, there is the worry that any offer of profit sharing with a donor may create an undue inducement for patients and other potential somatic cell providers to give biopsies for iPS cell derivations. Generally speaking, an undue inducement is defined as an offer of a reward so irresistible that it blinds individuals to the disadvantages and risks involved in a proposed research activity (Emanuel 2004). Undue inducements can threaten voluntary informed consent if they distract and cloud potential donors' thinking about their own well-being. Added to this is the further consequentialist warning that profit sharing with somatic cell donors may promote the commodification of human body parts for research and medical treatment (Dickenson 2008).

Both of these consequentialist arguments are rebuttable, however. Concerns very similar to these have already been raised in the area of egg-provider compensation for SCNT research, and I have argued extensively elsewhere that research regulators can reasonably address, as they have for decades, people's concerns about undue inducement and commodification while allowing fair compensation for a research volunteer's time, effort, and inconvenience (Hyun 2006b; 2011b).

It is also worth pointing out that, in the case of profit sharing with somatic cell donors, the ethical dangers of undue inducement are far less serious than they may be for SCNT egg providers. The physical risks involved in somatic cell donation are practically nonexistent; and although informational risks do exist (as discussed previously in this chapter), these can be managed through proper privacy protections. What exactly is there left for us to be worried about concerning the possible undue inducement of somatic cell donors?

Some may argue that permitting royalty payments for somatic cell donors would introduce financial incentives into the decision-making processes of future somatic cell providers. Such financial motivations would sully what should remain a pure, altruistically motivated act to support stem cell research. But others may respond that donor motivations can often be complex and multifaceted. Individuals in the real world might decide to offer their somatic cells to stem cell science for personal and charitable reasons. It would be naive to demand that all donors be driven only by selfless motives. If the argument is that it is ethically wrong somehow for research donors to be motivated in part by financial considerations, then this argument would also seem to apply to others who stand to gain financially from the commercial development of iPS cell and SCNT applications, such as the other parties listed previously. Why should somatic cell donors be the only altruistically motivated research enablers in the bunch?

It appears on further reflection that the undue inducement worry about somatic cell donors is really at heart a worry about the commodification of human body cells for stem cell derivations and commercial applications. If this is the more accurate diagnosis of the issue, then we must admit that we are already in the throes of this critic's feared state of affairs. It is the case that disease-specific stem cells are the object of much commercial interest. The commodification of human body cells and their pluripotent progeny has already begun. The question we must ask now, in light of this fact, is whether somatic cell donors have a right to be included anywhere along this money-making pipeline.

Our fuller diagnosis of the ethical issue here may turn out to be even more worrisome for some critics. Less adventurous spirits may wring their hands with the worry that iPS cell and other reprogramming technologies have set us on a path toward a dystopian future, where human biological materials come to be widely viewed as plastic instruments to be willfully engineered and sold for industrial purposes. It could be held that, in this dystopian future, many of our fundamental beliefs about our place in the natural order would be undermined if we allow human biological materials to be so heavily manipulated and exchanged for practical and commercial uses.

Others may not be very moved by these consequentialist alarm bells. First, the causal link between the commodification of human cells today and the long-term corrosion of how we view ourselves and our relation to science is wildly speculative at best. Even if we assume our activities now can change how people later think about the body and the nature of the social relationships supporting science, it is another claim altogether that this would be a change necessarily for the worse. Second, these fears may selectively ignore the counterbalancing possible benefits of cellular reprogramming – for example, the development of more effective interventions for patients and the reduction of physical risks to clinical trials volunteers. Gazing into their crystal balls, dystopian critics are far more likely to see reflections of their own fears, rather than a prescient view of an inevitable future. This is partly the problem with consequentialist moral reasoning. One gloomy crystal ball gazer can always be doubted by another gazer who is more optimistic in what he or she sees, and vice versa. While consequentialist moral prognosticators of both stripes debate and rebut each other's arguments, the question still remains whether somatic cell donors have a right to commercial royalties. This question gets complicated further by the uncertainties I raised previously regarding whether original donors have a moral claim to control what happens to derived stem cell lines. These interrelated sets of questions must be addressed by anyone interested in the moral rights of original donors.

## Conclusion

Practical research ethics as it pertains to the governance of stem cell research is an evolving area. Federal rules regarding biomedical research on human subjects aid our thinking to a certain extent, especially surrounding the issue of informational risk, but we need a set of much more stem cell–specific guidelines and regulations if we want to exert more direct ethical control over the full array of stem cell research activities. An SCRO committee oversight was designed to help in this endeavor, but even this approach is limited. I have identified in this chapter a series of important issues relating to the practical ethical conduct of stem cell research that seems to go beyond the powers of an SCRO committee. It is not clear what the correct approaches ought to be to address these emerging questions; neither is it clear exactly who is responsible for resolving them. Is it the investigators, the IRB, the SCRO committee, or someone else? These emerging issues involve philosophical questions about people's rights and their ontological connections to stem cell research materials. Anyone who tackles these philosophically rooted practical dilemmas must work within proper channels to ensure that resulting policies have institutional legitimacy. In the meantime, I fear that a kind of inertia in ethics and policy may begin to build while bioethicists and regulators wonder exactly who is responsible for taking on these issues and on what authority. In Chapter 5 I examine one area in which at least some open questions about stem cell regulatory reach and authority have been addressed, namely stem cell–based animal research.

# 5

# Pegasus and the Chimera

## *Stem Cell–Based Animal Research*

Chimera research is a common type of animal research used to advance stem cell science and many other areas of biomedicine. Biologically, chimeras are organisms that are composed of genetically distinct cells originating from two or more zygotes, or the imperfect equivalents thereof, such as parthenotes and SCNT embryolike constructs (Behringer 2007; Hyun et al. 2007). Unlike hybrids, which are produced by uniting the sex cells of two different species of plants or animals (wherein *each cell* contains the resulting new mixture of DNA – as is the case with grapefruit and mules), chimeric organisms are comprised of coexisting populations of cells with genes from different animal sources.

The term *chimera* comes from classical mythology. The Chimera, as described in Homer's *Iliad*, was a fire-breathing monster composed of the head of a lion, the body of a goat, and the tail of a serpent. The Chimera was, in essence, a patchwork of different animals. Given its patchwork nature, the Chimera lacked species integrity; and its physical capabilities were new and unpredictable.

Like the mythical Chimera, biological chimeras can be comprised of different species. They can also be comprised of members of the same species. For example, human pregnancies produce a mild form of chimerism that persists in mothers for decades after the fetus' progenitor blood cells have passed through the placenta (Bianchi et al. 1996). Human-to-human chimeras also occur naturally when two complete human zygotes fuse together during a very early developmental stage, prior to implantation in the womb. On rare occasions where the chimeric embryo proceeds to gestation, the resulting fetus is composed of cells from the two original embryos. More commonly, however, human-to-human chimeras result from clinical treatments for disease – the most obvious examples being the recipients of whole organ transplantation.

Hematopoietic stem cell transplantations for leukemia can also create chimeric humans when patients receive bone marrow transplants from a donor source. A new, more acute form of human chimerism is under development that results when a patient receives a hematopoietic stem cell transplant along with a grafted organ (e.g., a kidney) from the same donor. This combination of organ and bone marrow transplantation has been used to condition organ transplant recipients' immune systems to accept donor organs with minimal need for immune-suppressive drugs (Kawai et al. 2008). As these quick examples suggest, human-to-human chimeras are created through acts of nature during human reproduction and by certain medical interventions. Suffice it to say, human-to-human chimeras walk among us, and readers should note that if additional stem cell–based therapies are developed using donor cells, the prevalence of patient human chimeras is likely to increase. These facts are not normally cause for any alarm, nor should they be.

By contrast, the prospect of human/nonhuman chimeras seems to evoke strong repugnance among many people, despite the fact that very few of us are likely ever to encounter an interspecies chimera. Unlike human-to-human chimeras, human/nonhuman chimeras do not walk among us; rather, they are confined to laboratories where they are used for a wide range of biomedical research. For the purposes of this chapter, I shall set human-to-human chimeras to the side and focus exclusively on human/nonhuman chimeras.

Human/nonhuman chimera research has become commonplace over the past several decades, in large part because of the scientific advantages it offers over nonchimeric animal research. Nonchimeric laboratory animals (typically rodents) are generated to mimic human diseases through selective breeding, genetic engineering, or by physical or chemical means, after which they are used to assess the effectiveness of new drug interventions and other novel therapies. However, these purpose-built laboratory animals usually do not closely replicate human biology. For this reason, nonchimeric animal models of human disease do not always provide the surest means to aid the development of new therapeutic protocols. To overcome these limitations, human-to-animal chimera research aims to introduce localized human cellular and biological characteristics into laboratory animals. Animal models of human disease composed specifically of localized human tissues of investigational interest can be studied for their human-specific biological processes without experimentation on human subjects during very early stages of translational research (Behringer 2007). In essence, the overarching purpose of human/nonhuman chimera research is to *biologically human-ize* research animals in order to study human processes without using living human subjects.

Stem cell scientists join this ongoing scientific tradition of chimera research in several ways. In basic stem cell research, for example, human/nonhuman chimeras are created when scientists ascertain the quality of pluripotent human stem cells by using a teratoma assay in immune-deficient mice (recall the discussions in Chapter 2). Human/nonhuman chimera experiments can also shed light on how human stem cells and their derivatives behave in a living organism and integrate into complex organ systems. In translational stem cell research, chimera experiments take place when multipotent human stem cells or the derivatives of human pluripotent stem cells are transferred into laboratory animals to assess the safety and efficacy of new stem cell–based interventions. The FDA now recommends preclinical proof-of-principle studies using at least two different animal models for all stem cell–based biological product developments (Halme and Kessler 2006). Therefore, human/nonhuman chimera research is practically unavoidable if basic stem cell research is to transition toward clinical applications in humans. Whether for basic or for translational stem cell research, human/nonhuman chimeric animals can be utilized to help broaden our understanding of stem cell behavior beyond the confines of the culture dish, but before stem cells are studied in humans.

Unfortunately, the broad scientific value of human/nonhuman chimera research might not be enough to justify it in the eyes of many observers. Some may worry that, in the process of biologically humanizing animals, scientists may inadvertently humanize animals in a moral sense. That is, by pursuing stem cell–based human/nonhuman chimera research, a chief fear is that researchers might end up creating new creatures with full or near-human moral status sufficient to make experimenting on them ethically problematic (Streiffer 2005). This concern goes beyond some people's more general objections to animal research. For many this is a separate concern that human/nonhuman chimera research may be ethically undesirable even if one accepts that animal research could be ethically justified in other biomedical areas. Other critics may worry that, rather than elevating human/nonhuman chimeras to an equal or close-to-human level of moral status, this type of interspecies blending is a moral abomination that denigrates our own human dignity (Kass 2002; Schulman 2008). In short, human/nonhuman chimera research might be attacked from opposite camps: one side arguing that the biological humanization of animals may lead to their moral humanization, thus elevating these new beings to a level of protected moral status not possessed by other types of laboratory animals, and another side arguing that the creation of biologically humanized research animals diminishes our own human dignity.

In this chapter and in Chapter 6, I assess these two types of ethical concerns and expose the assumptions upon which they each seem to be based. In doing so, I propose a series of refinements to the worries outlined in the preceding text – refinements that may shed light on ultimately where our moral attention ought to be placed regarding stem cell–based chimera research.

## Chimeras – Past, Present, and Future

*Past Chimeras*

The original Chimera was a violent monster that terrorized the ancient Greeks. She was finally dispatched by the mortal Bellerophon, with the help of Pegasus and Athena's golden bridle. I suggested in Chapter 1 that the Chimera myth is a tale about the dangers of hubris and the use of transformative technologies for selfish ends, not a lesson about the intrinsic evils posed by the existence of mixed animals per se. Pegasus was, after all, also a chimeric animal, but a noble and admired creature, one that was said to have been used by Bellerophon numerous times for the benefit of the ancient Greeks (Hamilton 1942).

Chimeric animals appear in the folk narratives of many other ancient cultures. Like Pegasus and the Chimera, these mixed animals typically serve as powerful cultural symbols of good and evil. However, grasping the intended moral meanings of these mythical chimeras from a cultural distance is no simple task. Narrative context is everything. Different cultures might present physically similar chimeras but imbue them with opposite moral qualities depending on their role within a broader system of traditions and religious beliefs. For example, in contrast to the Greek Chimera, the Chinese Chimera Qilin was associated with the Confucian values of compassion and kindness and was said to appear only during times of peace and prosperity (Paludan 1981). The Egyptian Sphinx, unlike the malevolent Greek Sphinx, was a benevolent guardian of temples and royal tombs. And like the great Egyptian Sphinx, numerous other human/nonhuman chimeras dominate the polytheism of ancient Egypt and convey a host of important social and religious meanings. As depicted famously in the *Book of the Dead*, Anubis, the half man, half jackal Egyptian god of mummification would weigh the hearts of the deceased against the feather of Ma'at to determine who could enter the realm of the dead. Only those with hearts lighter than the feather (the lighthearted) would be allowed to enter the afterworld. The funerary deity Ammit – composed of a crocodile, lion, and hippopotamus – would devour the hearts of the unworthy. Historically, as these and many other examples suggest, chimeric creatures and deities held an important role within central cultural narratives and religious traditions, especially those dealing with humankind's perpetual anxieties, such as our loss of control and our own mortality.

The preceding observation – that mythical chimeras embodied either good or evil qualities and helped mediate people's hopes and fears of the unknown – is a fact that has illuminating implications for our discussion of stem cell–based chimera research. As the French anthropologist Claude Lévi-Strauss once observed, the myths of various cultures commonly begin with a presentation of opposing binary elements (good and evil, life and death, the natural and the supernatural, etc.) that are later resolved within the story to restore a sense of order to a seemingly arbitrary and unpredictable world (Lévi-Strauss 1963). Following Lévi-Strauss, I believe the vital lessons of all chimera mythologies lie in this eventual resolution of binary elements, and not in the initial acknowledgment that such unsettling binaries may exist. Readers should note that the Greek Chimera myth, the myth from which our term *chimera research* draws its origins, follows the binary patterns of good and evil, heaven and earth, control and chaos – embodied by Pegasus and the Chimera. To look only to the Chimera, that is, only one-half of these binaries, is erroneous because one may lose sight of the eventual resolution of the Chimera story and therefore the myth's fundamental lesson. Context matters for the purposes of moral instruction and assessment. In stem cell research, the binaries of life and death, health and disease, human and nonhuman are at play, and we need to attend to both halves of these dualities if we are to assess what moral conclusions might be drawn from attempts at their resolution through research.

Importantly, myths seem to offer other purposes besides providing a psychological resolution to people's anxiety-provoking binaries. Like Claude Lévi-Strauss, the American mythologist Joseph Campbell also analyzed commonalities underlying the world's mythologies, except he further theorized that myths tend to provide societies with at least four different functions: (1) a metaphysical, mystical function expressing one's awe of the universe; (2) a protoscientific cosmological function explaining why the natural world exists as it does; (3) a sociological function validating existing traditions and social institutions; and (4) a pedagogical function instructing individuals how to navigate themselves through different stages of life (Campbell 1991). If Campbell's analyses are correct, then we can conclude that chimera mythologies have also provided civilizations with one or more of these functions.

Today many, if not all, of these various functions of mythologies seem to have been co-opted by science, at least within most technologically advanced societies. Instead of mystical, protoscientific explanations of natural phenomena, we now have scientific, data-based explanations of our physical, biological, and social worlds. Instead of having our sense of metaphysical awe of the universe expressed through the telling of myths, we have grandiose, paradigm-shifting discoveries that equally convey our expansive sense of wonder.[1] One might even begin to suspect at this point that – for modern man – science is a kind of mythology that serves the same social functions that Lévi-Strauss and Campbell had previously hypothesized. This is an intriguing thought, but I would like to set it aside for the moment and focus more narrowly on the possibility that the sociological distinction between mythology and science could be blurred even further when the public is confronted with real-life biological analogues to mythical chimeras. The problem might be that, without any contextual knowledge of how to resolve the binary contradictions underscored by chimera research, the public might be left only with its initial impressions of perceived unsettling binaries, such as the human and the nonhuman, the natural and the unnatural, the person and the animal. And if science does not succeed in assuming the role that mythologies have had in resolving people's resulting anxieties, then, in these situations, one cannot help but suspect that ancient folk understandings and mystical beliefs about "essential animal natures" might begin to enter unconsciously into people's assessments of chimera research. Biological mixtures of humans and animals may inspire dreaded thoughts about what else this mixture might entail when human nature is combined with folk ideas of animal dispositions – that is, with the sloth of the pig, the sneakiness of the rat, or the villainy of the snake, and so forth.

The fact that chimera research is named after the Greek Chimera may do little to discourage people's mythological thinking and folk

---

[1] I am told by many reproductive and developmental biologists that, rather than dampening their awe of life processes, the discoveries of their respective fields do nothing but augment it.

beliefs from creeping into their thoughts about this controversial area of stem cell science. Why this tendency might exist I cannot explain, except to offer the tentative notion that this may be a deep-rooted, almost primeval human response. Others have touched on this point much more eloquently. Joseph Campbell was a close personal friend of the novelist John Steinbeck and the marine biologist Ed Ricketts. Perhaps inspired by Campbell's work, Steinbeck and Ricketts once wrote very movingly on the propensity of seafarers to believe in mythological sea creatures:

> [W]e have thought how the human fetus has, at one stage of its development, vestigial gill-slits. If the gills are a component of the developing human, it is not unreasonable to suppose a parallel or concurrent mind or psyche development. If there be a life-memory strong enough to leave its symbol in vestigial gills, the preponderantly aquatic symbols in the individual unconscious might well be indications of a group psyche-memory which is the foundation of the whole unconscious. And what things must be there, what monsters, what enemies, what fear of dark and pressure, and of prey! There are numbers of examples wherein even invertebrates seem to remember and to react to stimuli no longer violent enough to cause the reaction. (Steinbeck and Ricketts 1941, 32)

To follow Steinbeck and Ricketts's suggestion a bit further, I surmise that there may exist, if one will pardon the metaphor, "vestigial organs of thought" that gently tug our thinking down ancient conceptual pathways when we are stimulated by questions of the extreme unknown. Although there may be no conclusive remedy for this protoscientific psychological tendency, I believe our best response is to remain aware of the pull that mythological thinking has on people's beliefs about chimera research and to expose this influence whenever it occurs. It is against this background, this collective "psyche-memory" produced from our vestigial organs of thought, where "monsters ... enemies ... fear of dark and pressure, and of prey" lurk, that the science of chimera research stands to be examined by critics and the public.

### Present Chimeras

Most laypersons seem to be completely unaware of the extent to which both human/nonhuman and animal-to-animal chimera studies have been, and continue to be, employed in an enormous range of biomedical research. For decades, chimera studies have taught researchers much about fundamental biological processes and have aided the development of many therapeutic interventions for patients.

Outside of stem cell research, most human/nonhuman chimeras are created when human somatic cells or tissues are grafted into immune-deficient animals. Traditionally, genetically engineered immune-deficient athymic (nude) mice have been used as hosts for human/nonhuman chimera studies because their T-cell deficiency mutations allow a high tolerance for many types of foreign tissues. Other sources of immune-deficient animal hosts include using fetal animals before their immune systems have fully matured and using immunosuppressive drugs on genetically unaltered (wild type) postnatal animals.

Before one rushes to judge the ethical propriety of creating chimeric laboratory animals, it is valuable to pause for a moment and consider some of the broader research contexts of chimera experiments. For example, it should be remembered that cancer researchers and patients have benefited tremendously from human/nonhuman chimera research. The advent of immune-deficient nude mice has enabled researchers to graft bits of human tumors into mice, effectively turning these chimeric mice into cancer patients whose human tumors can be studied and screened with drugs (Behringer 2007). AIDS researchers and persons living with HIV have also benefited enormously from mouse models of the human immune system (the SCID-hu mouse), which are created when human lymphoid tissues are transplanted into immune-deficient mice to reconstitute distinct elements of the human immune system. By turning SCID-hu mice into HIV+ patients through direct inoculation of the HIV virus, researchers can test new antiviral drug interventions on laboratory animals that approximate the human condition before moving to human clinical trials (Bonyhadi and Kaneshima 1997).

Some observers may point out, however, that transferring diseased human tissues into immune-deficient rodents, or even swapping a mouse's immune system with a human one, is ethically unremarkable, because this type of chimerism is limited to anatomical sites that have no obvious bearing on a creature's moral status and so does not blur the lines between human and nonhuman in an ethically troubling way. By their lights, what is more worrisome is chimerism to an extreme degree, where the presence of human cells pervades throughout the animal host including, importantly, its CNS.

Critics may warn that acute human/nonhuman chimerism is made possible through the use of human multipotent and pluripotent stem cells.[2]

---

[2] I do not mean to suggest here that acute chimerism is possible *only* through the use of stem cells. E.g., acute chimerism can occur when two genetically distinct eight-cell

As background, it should be noted that the overall degree of human/nonhuman chimerism is believed to be determined by variables such as the type and number of human stem cells transplanted, the species and developmental stage of the host animal, and the anatomical location of the animal host where the stem cells are transferred (Lensch et al. 2007). When human pluripotent or multipotent stem cells are transplanted into a postnatal animal, it is unlikely that either type of stem cells will integrate significantly into the animal's existing biological structures during such a late stage of their development. If, however, pluripotent human stem cells are introduced into an embryonic or fetal animal host and allowed to develop in a reproductive context, such as a uterus, then the fractional percentage of differentiating human cells and the degree of human physiological integration in the developing animal host may turn out to be quite high, especially if there is little evolutionary distance between the animal species used and humans (Lensch et al. 2007). In light of this background, one might argue that, unlike the type of chimera studies used in cancer and AIDS research, stem cell–based chimera studies present a special case of chimera research that deserves close ethical scrutiny because of its potential to produce extreme degrees of human/nonhuman chimerism.

But what exactly is so troubling about acute human/nonhuman chimerism? I believe the real underlying ethical concern is not acute chimerism per se but rather what acute chimerism might imply about the resulting neurological humanization of the animal.[3] Most commentators have focused their discussions on acute neurological chimerism, which might occur when human pluripotent stem cells are transferred into

---

embryos are pushed together in a tissue culture after their outer *zona pellucidae* have been removed, resulting in an aggregation chimera. This aggregation chimera is formed prior to the blastocyst stage, and therefore it is not comprised of stem cells; rather, it later gives rise to genetically distinct precursor cells, which, if the aggregation embryo is implanted, go on to form an acutely chimeric fetus. To my knowledge, aggregation chimeras have not been created in the lab using human eight-cell embryos. Certainly the scientific value of this type of experiment would be very low, because we already know that early stage human embryos can aggregate together to form a chimera and implant in the womb, as so happens in cases of naturally occurring human-to-human chimeras. I discuss later in this chapter acute human/nonhuman chimerism using early stage embryos.

[3] Some critics may still have ethical objections to human/nonhuman chimera research if acute chimeras had no human contributions to the CNS and yet had bodies that were comprised of a majority of human cells. Robert Streiffer (2005) deftly deals with this "human appearance" objection to chimera research, and I refer readers to that discussion in his article.

early stage animal embryos, which are then gestated, or when large numbers of human multipotent or pluripotent stem cells or their derivatives are grafted into the CNSs of postnatal animal hosts (Greene et al. 2005; Karpowicz et al. 2004). Neurological human/nonhuman chimeras may be especially problematic for people who believe that the human brain is the locus of our unique moral characteristics. For those who maintain this view, the development of large amounts of human neurological matter in nonhuman animal brains may warrant concerns about the emergence of morally relevant mental properties in chimeric animals.

A cursory survey of some notable stem cell–based chimera studies may suggest that these special concerns are justified. For example, a group of Israeli scientists succeeded in creating human-chick chimeras by transferring one hundred to two hundred hES cells into one-and-a-half- and two-day-old chick embryos, wherein the hES cells survived, differentiated, and penetrated the host nervous system after one to five days of incubation. From this study the researchers concluded that chick embryos might serve as an easily accessible *in ovo* (in egg) system to study the biological development of hES cells (Goldstein et al. 2002). Another group of researchers at the Salk Institute reported that they had injected ten[5] hES cells into the brain ventricles of fetal mice to see if these human stem cells could differentiate successfully into functioning human neurons and integrate into the adult mouse forebrain. This experiment worked, leading the researchers to surmise that this neurological human-mouse chimeric model could aid the study of human neural development in a living organism (Muotri et al. 2005). A year later, a group at Rockefeller University injected clumps of ten to fifteen hES cells into preimplantation mouse blastocysts to test whether hES cells could incorporate into mouse embryos. Twenty-eight hES cell-mouse chimeric blastocysts were transferred into mouse uteruses and allowed to develop for five days. Upon collection and examination, four of these embryos had some hES cell–derived cells, leading the study authors to propose that hES cell development can be reconciled on rare occasions with mouse embryo development (James et al. 2006). Perhaps most controversially, human-monkey neurological chimeras were created in 2001 by a team led out of Harvard, where researchers transplanted approximately $2 \times 10^7$ human neural stem cells into the lateral brain ventricles of three fetal bonnet monkeys. The aim of this experiment was to use traceable human neural stem cells to ascertain whether the multiple populations of neural stem cells distributed throughout various regions of the CNS all originate from the same cell lineage or whether they represent unique pools of cells. The results of this human-monkey chimera experiment suggested that neural stem cells found throughout the CNS all originate from a common neural stem cell source very early in development. An analysis of host fetal monkey brains one month after transplantation showed the presence of human neurons and glial and undifferentiated human neural stem cells (Ourednik et al. 2001).

Some readers will look at these stem cell–based chimera studies with fascinated interest, while others will look at them in abject horror. A few points of qualification are in order here to help quell people's enthusiasm and disgust.

First, the actual degrees of human/nonhuman chimerism produced by the preceding studies were quite slight. In the Israeli study, less than half of the chimeric chick embryos survived to five days posttransplantation, and of those that did survive this brief incubation period, only very minute quantities of human cells could be detected. The Salk Institute study produced fetal human-mouse neurological chimeras that had on average less than 0.1 percent human brain cells. The Rockefeller University team detected derivatives of hES cells in very small quantities in four of the twenty-eight mouse embryos after direct injection at the blastocyst stage. Three of these chimeric embryos were developmentally aberrant, while the fourth one, which was less aberrant than the others, contained only ten cells derived from hES cells.[4] The Harvard team detected derivatives of human neural stem cells in each of the three chimeric fetal bonnet monkeys, at an average of about ten[5] human-derived cells per monkey brain. Interestingly, however, only 7 to 8 percent of these cells were human neurons, while the remaining quantity was comprised of human neural support cells (80% astrocytes and 12% oligodendrocytes).

Perhaps the limited chimerism evidenced in these studies could be explained in part by the short time periods in which the chimeric embryos and fetuses were allowed to develop and by the differences in developmental timing between human and nonhuman cells. Regardless of the specific reason, an important qualification to consider is that researchers did not produce acute human/nonhuman neurological chimeras despite the fact that they transferred human cells into embryonic and

---

[4] The study authors noted, however, that these ten human cells, which were detected by their green fluorescent protein markers, could have been the result of cell fusion with mouse cells rather than being bona fide derivatives of the green-tagged hES cells (James et al. 2006).

fetal animal hosts – one of the methodologies most feared by chimera research critics. One lesson to draw from these cases is that stem cell researchers can use early stage animal hosts to obtain new results without necessarily producing extreme neurological chimeras.

This leads us to our second important qualification. That is that the biological context into which human stem cells and their derivatives are placed has a significant influence on their cellular behavior. Biological context matters a great deal. Human cells that survive, develop, and pro-liferate in an animal host are heavily modulated and influenced by the animal's microenvironment. For example, the Salk Institute research-ers who conducted the chimeric mouse brain study observed that the human-derived neurons seemed to respond to local differentiation sig-nals in the developing mouse and, as a result of this, acquired physical characteristics and functions similar to the host's mouse neurons (Muotri et al. 2005). The Israeli scientists noted that hES cells transplanted directly into chick embryos were heavily modulated in their develop-ment by the host embryonic environment (Goldstein et al. 2002).

Observations such as these support a prevalent view among devel-opmental biologists that human stem cells and their derivatives do not simply run on "auto-pilot."[5] Rather, their development is an integrative process of cell responses and interactions within a given biological envi-ronment. When transplanted into animals, human stem cells do not carry with them an Aristotelian-like deterministic agency or a biologi-cal "human essence." This is true whether we are talking about human tumors or immune systems transplanted into immune-deficient rodents, or whether we are talking about human stem cells and their derivatives transferred into animal embryos and fetuses.

As a case in point, past mouse experiments designed specifically to produce functioning human/mouse chimeric brains did not establish host brain functions beyond control levels in nonchimeric mice (Lensch et al. 2007). Instead, the human neurons and support cells that devel-oped in mouse hosts did so by responding to and integrating with exist-ing mouse neural structures, rather than directing the hosts to develop a humanlike brain architecture (Brustle et al. 1998; Flax et al. 1998; Kerr et al. 2003; Mueller et al. 2005; Nistor et al. 2005; Tabar et al. 2005). A simple analogy might help underscore this important idea.[6] We know

[5] I thank Willy Lensch for raising this excellent point.
[6] This analogy comes from Hank Greely (Shreeve 2005), which I have modified slightly here.

that transferring electrical wires from a cathedral into a gas station does not thereby turn that gas station into a cathedral. The electrical wires do not carry with them the cathedral's architectural blueprint or any other qualities that make it a cathedral. All we can say is that the gas station's new wires came from a cathedral. Much the same can be said about human neural cells. They are human cells in so far as they came from a human source; they do not carry with them any sort of deterministic human biological agency, not even if they are derived from human pluripotent stem cells.[7]

Some critics have argued that these admissions militate against the scientific rationale for conducting stem cell–based chimera studies (Baylis and Fenton 2007). If these experiments do not give us an unadulterated view of human biological processes as they would occur in real human bodies, then why do them at all? I believe the best response to this question is to recognize that chimera studies give us a partial yet illuminating view of human processes. Although chimeric animal systems are not exactly identical to a fully realized human biology, their use is at least more informative than the use of *in vitro* studies solely, especially considering the fact that three-dimensional niche structures are important for the dynamics of stem cell behavior (see Chapter 2). We just have to be very careful about the scientific interpretations we might justifiably draw from human/nonhuman chimera studies.

The third qualification I wish to point out is that each of the aforementioned chimera studies was conducted in accordance with strict institutional requirements for animal research, which include among these conditions a defined experimental endpoint and a humane method for euthanizing the study animals. I elaborate on these and other animal research requirements in the next section, but it is worth briefly noting here that, due to biosafety regulations, no human/nonhuman chimera studies conducted at institutions accredited for animal research can permit research animals to roam free at the conclusion of the study. This is why no human/nonhuman chimeras walk among us, and one reason why some people are so dismayed by animal research – because these studies normally conclude with the termination and histological examination of laboratory animals.

---

[7] The same can be said for human genes. E.g., researchers transferred a human eye gene into a mutant mouse that lacked the gene for mouse eyes. This human-eye-gene transfer produced in the mouse not a human eye, but a mouse eye. A human eye gene rescues a mouse eye when placed into a murine biological context (Schedl et al. 1996).

*Future Chimeras*

As biomedical researchers attempt to develop new stem cell–based therapies for patients, they will first have to conduct safety and proof-of-principle studies in animal models of human disease. These animal models will have to provide reasonable approximations of human medical conditions. Depending on the disease or injury in question, some researchers may wish to use host animals that are closer to the size and/or physiology of humans, such as pigs or nonhuman primates, not rodents or chicks, which are quite remote physically from humans.

In addition to their size advantages, larger animal species may have brain structures, cranial capacities, life spans, and developmental rates that are more proximate to humans, making them better models for human neurological disorders. Whether through controlled injury, early developmental-stage human/nonhuman chimerization, or by chemical means, the brains of large laboratory animals would have to be altered to mimic human neural pathologies. After the relevant neurological alteration is in place, a human stem cell–based cellular therapy of interest will have to be administered at a clinically relevant dose, which is likely to be quite high. Thus the resulting degree of human/nonhuman neurological chimerism might be substantial – at least if investigators are hopeful of producing clinically significant results, such as the restoration of a brain function or the prevention of neurological degradation.

As the Harvard primate/human neural stem cell study showed, the migration, differentiation, and integration of human neural cells is achievable in developing old-world primate brains, making it reasonable to suppose that the creation of disease-modeled human/primate chimeric brains and the integration of human stem cell–based therapeutic cells are in principle possible in nonhuman primates. This is a potential future direction for human/nonhuman stem cell–based chimera research, and it is for many observers the most controversial. Unlike chimera studies involving rodent or chick hosts, it is far less certain what will happen developmentally if researchers attempt to chimerize the brains of animal species that are evolutionarily closer to humans.

It is unknown where stem cell–based translational chimera research will take us in the future. But without a practical and philosophical ethical framework to help us address these uncertainties, people's mythological fears and anxieties could end up driving the decisions around this new area of stem cell science. In the next section I explain how human/nonhuman chimera research is overseen at the level of practical research ethics, beginning with live animal research and then moving briefly to *in vitro* embryo studies. Then in Chapter 6 I revisit the chief ethical concerns surrounding human/nonhuman neurological chimera studies, specifically those involving large animal species similar to man. I conclude that chapter by raising a number of unresolved philosophical issues that must be explored before any definitive conclusions can be drawn concerning the ethics of creating acute human/nonhuman neurological chimeras.

## Chimera Research Oversight

All stem cell–based chimera research involving postnatal live animals is subject to institutional and legal regulations for animal research. Thus, if we are to get a complete picture of chimera research oversight at the practical research ethics level, we must start with the regulatory requirements for animal research.

Scientific and ethical standards for animal research are well defined in laws, international and national guidance documents, and international standards for voluntary accreditation (e.g., the Association for Assessment and Accreditation of Laboratory Care International), as well as in the academic literature (National Research Council 1996; Orlans 1993; Rollin and Kesel 1990). In the United States, all animal research must be reviewed and approved by an independent scientific and ethics board called an IACUC. All IACUCs and their equivalent review committees abroad utilize the following standards: (1) the proposed animal research must have substantial scientific merit, and there must be no scientifically acceptable alternative method for answering the research question; (2) the research must be conducted in appropriate facilities by well-trained staff, including veterinarians qualified to care for the species involved; (3) the lowest statistically significant number of animals must be used, without undue pain and stress, and with environmental enrichment appropriate for the species; (4) experimental endpoints must be clearly defined, and euthanasia methods must be humane and veterinarian approved; and (5) ongoing monitoring of approved animal research shall be conducted by the review committee, which has the power to terminate or suspend studies (National Research Council 1996). All of these standards must be upheld before any new animal research proposal can commence. And all top-tier scientific journals require assurance that researchers have met IACUC standards before their work can be published.

In addition to considerations of scientific merit and statistical sample size – which both relate to the scientific integrity requirement of research ethics (see Chapter 3) – the primary focus of animal research oversight is to ensure as much as possible that species-specific animal welfare considerations are responsibly upheld by animal researchers and their institutions. Animal welfare considerations tend to focus primarily on the likelihood of pain, anxiety, and/or suffering experienced by laboratory animals during the course of a study. Importantly, the degree of animal welfare at stake will depend on the physical and mental complexity of the animal, so that a study involving amphibians will have less complicated animal welfare requirements than a mouse study, and a mouse study less complicated requirements than a study involving pigs, and so forth. Because more complex animals may experience greater degrees of pain and suffering, animal research oversight committees require that the "lowest" possible species be used to answer the research question and that appropriate sedation or anesthesia be used to minimize possible discomfort and distress.

Besides meeting IACUC standards for animal research, all stem cell–based chimera research must also be approved by an SCRO committee (see Chapter 4). The requirement for SCRO committee review is stipulated by American and international stem cell–specific research guidelines (ISSCR 2006; National Academy of Sciences 2005). The stated purpose of SCRO review of chimera research is to supplement, not duplicate, IACUC oversight. However, these stem cell research guidelines do not explain in much detail what SCRO committees are supposed to add to the animal research oversight process.

To help fill this void, the Ethics and Public Policy Committee of the ISSCR authored an advisory report outlining its stem cell–specific recommendations for the SCRO review of chimera research (Hyun et al. 2007). The committee presented its recommendations in generally applicable terms, because diverse institutions and international settings may impose their own additional standards for animal research, requiring investigators and reviewers to exercise their best professional judgment in each individual case.

Among the committee's key recommendations (which I merely summarize here) is the proposal that SCRO review should build on existing IACUC standards for animal welfare in scientific research. That is, SCRO committees should add additional ethical standards only if something specific to stem cell research makes it necessary to do so.

Let us consider a primary example of this approach. Current IACUC evaluations of animal welfare are conducted at a species-specific level. This species-specific approach, however, may still leave open special questions for neurological human/nonhuman stem cell–based chimeras, because such chimerism may (theoretically) pose a change in sentience or behavior from nonchimerized animals. Past experience with genetically altered laboratory animals has shown that reasonable caution might be warranted if genetic changes carry the potential to produce new behaviors and especially new defects and deficits. Best practices today dictate that research involving genetically modified animals must involve the following: (1) the establishment of baseline animal data; (2) ongoing data collection during research concerning any deviation from the norms of species-typical animals; (3) the use of small pilot studies to ascertain any welfare changes in modified animals; and (4) ongoing monitoring and reporting to oversight committees authorized to decide the need for protocol changes and the withdrawal of animal subjects (Hyun et al. 2007).

These four steps aim to help minimize the occurrence of unexpected distress and suffering in genetically modified animals. Contrary to what many laypersons may believe, such bioengineered animals are not usually enhanced above normal species functioning. Rather, the far more typical outcome of genetically modifying research animals is their lower levels of physical functioning (e.g., mouse models of cystic fibrosis).

The ISSCR Ethics and Public Policy Committee's report effectively extends these four steps to the SCRO review of human/nonhuman chimera research. The SCRO committees must include experts in stem cell and developmental biology who can assess the likely developmental trajectories produced when signaling modules from different species are mixed during the course of a proposed chimera experiment, taking into account the epigenetic context of regulation in which the mixed cells are going to be deployed. As with genetically modified research animals, SCRO committees ought to require that a baseline of normal animal data be created before chimera experimentation can be permitted. These data might include behavioral and other necessary information for animal welfare, such as hormonal data related to indicators of stress and anxiety. Such baseline data must be grounded in rigorous scientific knowledge or reasonable inferences, not speculative notions about animal mental states and experiences that are contrary to known brain functional requirements and accepted scientific facts.

The committee report also recommends that researchers use small pilot studies to produce initial data on chimeric animals to monitor and describe any deviations from normal behaviors – the same sort of steps researchers would employ for the use of new, genetically modified animals. Contrary to the fears of many opponents of human/nonhuman chimera research, the Ethics and Public Policy Committee was far less concerned about the possibility of "enhanced" humanlike chimeric animals springing into existence in stem cell laboratories. Instead, the committee was much more mindful of the very real possibility (based on experience with transgenic and genetically modified animals) that chimeric research animals will exhibit interrupted equilibria and major biological deficiencies, which would call into action a most diligent application of animal welfare principles.

In summary, the ISSCR chimera report recommends that stem cell investigators, animal research regulators, and SCRO committees extend existing animal welfare standards – in particular, standards for the oversight of heavily modified animals – to cover new human/nonhuman chimeric research animals in a careful, stepwise fashion.

The committee arrived at this series of recommendations after careful consideration of the objections typically mounted against human/nonhuman chimera research. For instance, the committee was not very concerned by the prospect of human chimeric embryo studies. Such research was deemed to be permissible as long as researchers follow ISSCR guidelines by not allowing chimeric preimplantation human host embryos to develop in culture for more than fourteen consecutive days, or beyond the appearance of the embryo's primitive streak, and by not implanting into a human or nonhuman primate uterus any embryo containing transplanted human pluripotent stem cells.[8] The first stipulation accepts that the moral status of a human or nonhuman host embryo up to fourteen days of development is not affected by its possible degree of chimerism. If it is ethically permissible to use entirely unchimerized human embryos for *in vitro* stem cell research, then it should be ethically permissible to use chimerized human or nonhuman host embryos for *in vitro* research. The second stipulation mentioned accepts that it would be ethically undesirable to implant a human/nonhuman chimeric embryo into a uterine environment capable of supporting its full

---

[8] Stem cell research guidelines issued by the NAS permit the transfer of human pluripotent stem cells into preimplantation blastocysts of any species except human and nonhuman primates.

gestation. This restriction is motivated by an interest in avoiding indiscriminate human/nonhuman chimerism, especially within a reproductive context that is very hard to predict and control. The restriction is not meant to prevent a more localized and scientifically controlled development of acute human/nonhuman chimeras. After all, American and international stem cell guidelines allow for the transfer of human pluripotent stem cells into nonhuman animals at their embryonic and fetal stages of development, where the chances of producing acute chimerism are high within localized animal structures. Similarly, the ISSCR Ethics and Public Policy Committee did not categorically advise against the possibility of creating acute human/nonhuman chimeras either in embryonic or later developmental stages. Instead, the report advises that scientifically justified research that may result in significantly humanized mental attributes in human/nonhuman chimeras, while not absolutely prohibited, must be subject to close monitoring and careful data collection pertinent to the welfare of animal subjects.

Finally, the committee was not persuaded by dignity arguments against human/nonhuman chimera research. Some commentators have suggested that chimera research could weaken the human/nonhuman boundary, thereby degrading our human dignity (Kass 2002; Schulman 2008). Similarly, NAS states in its stem cell research guidelines that:

> Research in which hES cells are introduced into nonhuman primate blastocysts ... should also not be conducted at this time. These kinds of studies could produce creatures in which the lines between human and nonhuman primates are blurred, a development that could threaten to undermine human dignity. (National Academy of Sciences 2005, 55)

Dignity arguments such as these are deeply flawed. The Ethics and Public Policy Committee recognized that human dignity is a multidimensional concept usually characterized by a set of valuable human capacities, such as the capacity for moral agency, self-consciousness, and high-level emotional and cognitive functions. Human dignity is not a property of human cells, but rather a property of whole human beings that is not diminished in the least if new creatures are created that might be said to share some of these capacities. Unlike relational properties, such as being rare or being unique, human dignity is not a kind of property that diminishes or runs out when it is ascribed to more individuals who may deserve a claim to it (Hyun et al. 2007).

I would like to bolster this last point with the following philosophical analysis. Regardless of the specific religious or cultural traditions from which one's notion of human dignity gets its source, human dignity should be understood by all of us as an intrinsic property of individuals, not an extrinsic property. An *intrinsic property* is defined in philosophy as a property that a thing has in virtue of the way that thing is. An extrinsic property is that which a thing has that depends on something else outside of itself being true (Lewis 1983). For example, my being male is an intrinsic property of me, while my being a parent is an extrinsic property. In the case of human dignity, philosophers widely agree that this is something a person possesses intrinsically, regardless of his or her social class, geographical location, cultural milieu, and the like. It is from this understanding of human dignity (as an intrinsic property of persons) that this notion packs so much political force in the rhetoric of international covenants, such as 1948 Universal Declaration of Human Rights. Human dignity is not something individuals leave at the customs counter when they cross national borders. It is something they carry with them at all times, wherever they are.

To argue that the creation of human/nonhuman chimeras threatens our human dignity is to view human dignity as an extrinsic property, one that can be affected by actions taking place away from us. But it is not an extrinsic property. It is an intrinsic property. Human dignity is violated only when undeserved harms are imposed directly onto one's self, such as torture, rape, or slavery. The "undermining of human dignity" argument against human/nonhuman chimera research – be it of an *in vitro*, embryonic, fetal, or postnatal nature – lacks philosophical coherence when critics claim that experiments taking place outside of ourselves, on a few laboratory animals in scientific research facilities, lessens in any way our own intrinsic properties. To make the claim that chimera research violates human dignity is, in my view, an affront to people whose dignity has truly been victimized, such as those ravaged by genocide, those starving in extreme poverty or famine, or patients in the throes of a degenerative neurological disorder like Huntington's disease. Thus, to avoid being politically glib and insensitive to true human suffering, and for the sake of our own philosophical coherence, we ought to abandon permanently the "undermining of human dignity" argument against chimera research.

## Conclusion

In light of the points summarized in the preceding text, the ISSCR Ethics and Public Policy Committee's recommendations seem to provide a workable framework for overseeing chimera research – building on and remaining consistent with IACUC animal welfare principles, but with added stem cell–specific expertise to consider the further developmental effects on animal welfare of human stem cell–based chimerism.

Some may wonder, however, whether these guidelines are sufficient to handle ethical concerns surrounding acute human/nonhuman neurological chimerism in large animal species, particularly nonhuman primates. It would appear that simply extending animal welfare principles to these types of acute neurological chimeras is not enough. For one, this approach still operates within the framework of animal research. But what if stem cell scientists end up producing acute neurological chimeras with a moral status that approximates or is equal to ours? What if, in the process of conducting stem cell–based animal research, scientists create new beings that are humanized not just biologically, but also morally? Would this still count as animal research, or would it end up being something else? And if it is something else, then should we allow it? How should we respond to these disturbing questions?

In the face of this uncertainty, some people may retreat to the dark corners of their subconscious and emerge with an inner visceral resistance to allow such research. Fear appears to be a common human response to the unknown. Again, the observations of other writers may be instructive of this human propensity.

The famed mythologist Edith Hamilton once explained that the classical myths, which still play upon people's imaginations today, were shaped during a time when few methodical distinctions were drawn between the real and the unreal. Of the poets who lived during this early human period, she wrote:

> The imagination was vividly alive and not checked by the reason, so that anyone in the woods might see through the trees a fleeing nymph, or bending over a clear pool to drink behold in the depths a naiad's face. (Hamilton 1942, 3)

But the poets may have overanimated their world with colors much brighter than those experienced by the common man. Hamilton concluded her dreamy train of thought with this harsh point:

> Nothing is clearer than the fact that primitive man ... is not and never has been a creature who peoples his world with bright fancies and lovely visions. Horrors lurked in the primeval forest, not nymphs and naiads. (Hamilton 1942, 4)

Like Hamilton's ancient poets, stem cell scientists are apt to see wonderful and captivating revelations in their work. But the lay public, like men hunting for survival in a primeval forest, may be much more attuned to unknown potential dangers. When faced with unfamiliar scientific proposals, their thoughts might pull habitually toward the prospect of a frightful Chimera rather than the elegant usefulness of a bridled Pegasus.

To help address these uncertainties, I consider in Chapter 6 what I call the "limit case" of human/nonhuman chimera research. Carefully reflecting on the limit case may offer some valuable heuristics. First, we can uncover through this process a series of hidden assumptions and presuppositions that, when exposed and disarmed, may help us reconcile our anxieties about acute neurological chimerism. And second, once we sharpen our thinking about the limit case, we may be better situated to clarify our thoughts on gradients of human/nonhuman chimera research falling below the limit level.

# 6

## The Limit Case

### *Acute Human/Nonhuman Neurological Chimerism*

Acute human/nonhuman neurological chimerism arguably might yield the most scientific utility if it is produced in large animal species that are already physiologically very similar to human beings. In view of this supposition, some may propose that the biologically ideal species for acute neurological chimera studies are large old-world monkeys and great apes. Their genetic proximity to us, larger cranial capacities, and more humanlike developmental rates might all better accommodate the chimeric development of a functional human brain–like architecture and thus could pose significant advantages over the use of small animals. It is for much of these same reasons, however, that many people are uncomfortable with the prospect of this type of chimera research. The fear is that acute neurological chimerism in nonhuman primates might render them not only much more biologically like us, but also far more morally comparable. In this chapter I explore these and other ethical concerns.

Others have written on the issue of acute human/nonhuman neurological chimerism, but none has analyzed this topic in the manner that I do in the following text. Phillip Karpowicz and colleagues (2004, 2005) argue that such experiments should be allowed, but only under the following conditions: (1) limiting the number of human cells transferred to the fewest necessary to achieve the research aim; (2) limiting the choice of host animal to the least morphologically and functionally related to humans as possible for the study; and (3) using only dissociated human cells, rather than postanatomical tissue transplants, in developing embryonic chimeras. Robert Streiffer (2005) recommends an early termination (abortion) policy on acutely chimeric human/nonhuman embryos before the formation of a cognitive system, or, in the absence of such a policy, a restriction on the transfer of human pluripotent stem cells into early stage developing animals. Mark Greene and colleagues (2005) recommend that review committees consider the following factors in considering the permissibility of human/nonhuman primate neural grafting experiments: the proportion of engrafted human cells, neural development, the species of nonhuman primate, brain size, the site of integration, and brain pathology. Greene and colleagues suggest that the review of neural grafting experiments should also involve data collection on any changes in cognitive function and behavior.

Notably, none of these reports explains exactly what reviewers and researchers ought to be seeking when looking for changes in chimeric animals toward more "humanlike" functions and behaviors. Streiffer comes closest by saying that the relevant enhancements would be "high-level" cognitive capacities, although he does not explain what this means and how one might look for these capacities in neurological chimeras. Thus I believe it is crucial that we pursue further exactly what "humanlike" characteristics we ought to identify as important in evaluating the ethical permissibility of acute neurological chimera studies, and whether it would be possible in practice to detect the emergence of these characteristics.

To help us toward these goals, I suggest we directly confront the limit case for human/nonhuman neurological chimerism. Because the limit case represents for many people the "worst-case scenario" for stem cell–based chimerism, it is worth our while to explore it in some detail. Some readers may find the discussions in this chapter to be abstract and arduous. It is important, however, for readers to persevere through this philosophical discourse. I believe a careful and persistent examination of the issues covered in the following text will help raise people's awareness of many important questions surrounding the ethics of acute neurological chimerism that have been, to the best of my knowledge, regrettably ignored in the bioethics literature.

## Setting Up the Limit Case

For the purposes of the limit case, I shall assume that the host animal is a prenatal old-world primate with large quantities of human stem cells or their direct derivatives transplanted directly into its developing brain. The (hypothetical) scientific goal of the limit case would be to gestate the resulting chimeric fetus to produce a postnatal research animal with a functioning, acutely chimeric human/nonhuman brain for disease modeling and/or proof-of-principle stem cell–based neurological interventions.[1]

To help focus our attention on the philosophical and ethical issues raised by the limit case, I shall conveniently set aside some important real-world issues and constraints. I will bring these points back for our consideration later, after we have analyzed the limit case in its more simplified form.

The first point I wish to bracket is the fact that the type of chimera research imagined here might not be permitted in many parts of the world given current and pending regulatory restrictions on the use of large old-world primates for invasive research.[2] For example, the United Kingdom permits scientific procedures to be carried out on old-world primates, such as rhesus monkeys, but it does not permit invasive research on great apes, such as chimpanzees. Only the United States and the West African state of Gabon allow invasive research on chimpanzees, with the vast majority of these studies centering on hepatitis-C vaccine development. The status of such research in the United States may soon change, however, because the U.S. Institute of Medicine (IOM) recently released a report advising the federal government that most invasive biomedical research on chimpanzees is not currently scientifically justified (Institute of Medicine 2011). This IOM report may drastically curtail the continuation of invasive chimpanzee research, because U.S. primate facilities rely on federal funding for their infrastructure and long-term primate care (Wadman 2011). For the purposes of the limit case, I shall assume that stem cell researchers have access to large nonhuman primates for invasive chimera studies.

Furthermore, I shall assume that the following conditions also hold true: (1) that large nonhuman primates are available to study investi-

---

[1] Note that the limit case would not violate ISSCR guidelines as long as human pluripotent stem cells or their direct derivatives are transplanted into the CNSs of very early fetal primates *in utero*. (The ISSCR guidelines prohibit transferring human stem cells into a preimplantation nonhuman primate embryo with the plan to transfer the resulting chimeric embryos into a nonhuman primate uterus.) Also note that I am excluding from the limit case attempts to chimerize a postnatal nonhuman primate brain with human pluripotent or multipotent stem cells or their direct derivatives. Attempts at postnatal acute neurological chimerism are not likely to result in an extensive integration of human cells into an already developed primate brain, much less redirect the brain to assume a more humanlike architecture.

[2] In 2008 Spain became the first country to grant human rights to the great apes. There are ongoing legislative debates in many parts of Europe, led by members of the Great Ape Project, concerning whether nonhuman primates ought to be afforded the status of persons.

gators in sufficient numbers to generate statistically meaningful results; (2) that the cost of using these complex animal models is not prohibitively expensive; (3) that there is no other way to answer the research question – that is, there are no other animal species with a greater evolutionary distance from us that can serve as appropriate hosts for the chimera study; and (4) that the developmental interactions between the derived human neural cells and the host primate's are indicative of what would happen in a fully human biological context. One may argue that, in the real world, most, if not all, of these suppositions are not likely to be realized, thus making the limit case, practically speaking, a nonstarter. I suspect that many of these practical arguments are valid, and I shall return to them at the end of this chapter. But for now I wish to focus our attention on the philosophical issues, which, if they come out ethically against the limit case, would provide additional strength to the practical arguments, or, in situations in which the practical constraints could be overcome, would stand as our only ethical defense.[3]

Finally, it must be acknowledged that many people are strongly against invasive nonhuman primate research, either because they are opposed to *all* animal research, or because they believe nonhuman primates possess a degree of moral status that makes their use in invasive animal research wrong. (Personally, I am very sympathetic to this latter view.) Such opponents would rate my call to examine the chimera limit case as entirely superfluous, because for them the limit case would fall under the category of unethical scientific experimentation. However, many researchers, regulators, and funders may not view the use of nonhuman primates in chimera research as ethically out-of-bounds. Therefore, I direct my limit case in the following text to those who believe that invasive nonhuman primate research is, in principle, ethically permissible, as long as active measures are taken to reduce or to eliminate animal pain and suffering during the course of research. For persons who maintain these permissive beliefs, the key question for them to consider is whether the acute neurological chimerism of nonhuman primates could ever raise their (presumably lower) moral status as sentient beings to a critical point at which invasive studies would become ethically impermissible.

[3] Furthermore, existing practical limitations in some locales for the prospect of large-scale nonhuman primate chimera studies may be absent in other locales, especially if private funding is available from parties interested in supporting the research. Thus it is important for us to soldier on with our consideration of the limit case.

## Searching for Factor X

My methodological approach to the limit case can be outlined as follows. In order to determine whether neurologically chimeric nonhuman primates could ever cross into the realm of our moral humanity, we would have to narrow our focus in the limit case to the type of enhancement or set of enhancements that would suffice to constitute this moral status upgrade. Let us call this philosophical task the search for Factor X. We begin by assuming *ex hypothesis* that nonhuman primates lack Factor X, while human beings have it. (It should be noted that Factor X does not have to be a single property; it may be, for all we know, a cluster of properties.) If nonhuman primates were to gain Factor X during the course of an acute human/nonneurological chimera study, then proponents of this type of research would have an ethical problem on their hands. Once we define what Factor X is, our next step would be to explain how we are to detect the presence of Factor X in chimeric laboratory animals. The first task – that of philosophically defining Factor X – is difficult enough. The second task – that of coming up with an empirical test for detecting Factor X in laboratory animals – may be just as difficult to realize, if not more so.

The prime candidate for Factor X appears to be some type of mental faculty or set of faculties, because people's concerns about acute human/nonhuman chimerism seem to boil down to worries about the moral consequences of greatly mingling the neurological biology of humans and animals. Readers will find this connection intuitive and obvious. However, readers should also realize how challenging it is to identify further what Factor X might be after we have made this initial categorical cut. What may initially appear to be a series of scientific inquiries proves on closer inspection to be an inherently philosophical undertaking. In our search for Factor X, we must traverse a conceptual landscape filled with competing philosophical ideas and value-laden choices over which empirical methodology to employ wherever empirical methodologies might come into play. That is to say, whenever measurements may be advisable to aid our thinking about the limit case, the choice over which kinds of measurements to employ is a theoretically driven decision. To substantiate this insight, let us consider the following progression of issues.

If Factor X is a mental faculty (or set of faculties) that human beings possess but normal, unchimerized nonhuman primates lack, then we should be able to narrow down the possible candidates for Factor X by comparing the normal mental faculties of nonhuman primates to the normal mental faculties of humans. Factor X, if it exists at all, would have to be found somewhere on the human side of the differences between the two. But locating it along the human divide of these differences is simply not enough. We also have to explain plausibly how Factor X supports a higher moral status in human beings. For example, let us suppose for the sake of argument that human beings can perceptually experience a particular shade of color that nonhuman primates cannot. This ability would count as a mental faculty that human beings have that nonhuman primates lack, but it surely would serve nothing to support a view that human beings therefore possess a higher moral status as a result of this. Not only must Factor X be a property present in humans but absent in nonhuman primates; it must also be morally important.

Many people would argue that moral status is cognitively based, so if we are looking for Factor X in the limit case, we need to look within the realm of human cognition. Human cognition is comprised of a wide set of mental faculties that includes perception, learning, memory, spatial awareness, communication, language, numeracy, causal reasoning, metacognition (thinking about thinking), and social cognition – for example, a theory of mind (an awareness of the existence of other minds) and self-consciousness (Andrews 2011). Animal cognition, by contrast, appears to be less involved, as it is believed to involve only perception, learning, memory, spatial awareness, and decision making (i.e., mental processes that generate adaptive or flexible behaviors in the face of change). In our limit case, neurologically chimeric nonhuman primates would gain the moral status enjoyed by humans only if they were to obtain human cognitive abilities through their biological chimerization. If we continue under the assumption that moral status is cognitively based and that Factor X amounts to one or more morally important forms of human cognition, we quickly run headlong into a thorny tangle of philosophical questions.

First, we may wonder whether the differences between human and nonhuman primate cognition are differences in *degree* or in *kind*. If they are differences in kind, then morally problematic neurological chimerism would have to amount to a true transformation in the way in which nonhuman primates think, not merely an improvement in what they are capable of doing. This would be a very high bar for neurological chimerism to have to pass before proponents of this research would need to start worrying about it.

There are good philosophical reasons for supposing that the cognitive differences between humans and nonhuman primates are differences in kind. Most contemporary philosophers of mind maintain that cognitive systems involve beliefs. Traditionally, beliefs are defined as mental representations that express propositional content (i.e., that such and such is or is not the case: that the cup is on the table; that the drink is no longer hot; and so forth). An alternative formulation identifies a belief as a propositional attitude – that is, as a mental state of having an attitude or opinion about a proposition or about a potential state of affairs in which that proposition is true (e.g., that the cup is on the table, and so forth). According to either of these philosophical definitions, beliefs are propositional. This is an important point for us to bear in mind because it may explain how beliefs about beliefs (second-order beliefs) and meta-cognition (thinking about thinking) are possible, that is, through the embedding of propositions within propositions. If the cognitive systems of nonhuman primates are similar in kind to human cognitive systems (albeit not realized to the same degree), then nonhuman primates must also have propositionally grounded beliefs. But what would it mean for nonhuman primates to have such beliefs?

Most philosophers would argue that, without language, nonhuman primates cannot have beliefs in the way that beliefs have traditionally been understood. Instead, nonhuman primates would have to have beliefs that are nonpropositional. What would this type of belief amount to? One possible view is that such beliefs are based on simple imagistic mental representations, such as nonlinguistic "maps" or "diagrams" of the external world (Camp 2009). If this is true, then nonhuman primates and humans would have cognitive systems that are different in kind, not degree. Importantly, one key point that comes out of this is that nonhuman primates would lack the ability to form second-order thoughts or have beliefs about their beliefs. This would pose serious constraints on the possibility that neurological chimerism could elevate the moral status of nonhuman primates by enhancing how they are able to think. Neurological chimerism would have to transform, not merely improve, nonhuman primates into becoming humanlike thinkers with propositional beliefs, all without the aid of language.

For many philosophers, however, having propositional beliefs without language is an impossibility (Davidson 1982). They maintain that having propositional beliefs requires cognitive agents to grasp the notion that beliefs can be either true or false. But in order to develop an understanding of truth and falsity, an individual needs to be able to communicate with others about their experiences of the world and compare their points of view. Thus, on this view, cognitive agents must be language users if they are to have propositional beliefs.

Some may insist that a few nonhuman primates have been able to use American Sign Language (ASL), thereby suggesting the possibility that nonhuman primates, especially the great apes, are capable of having humanlike propositional beliefs. These species have included a gorilla (Patterson 1978), some chimpanzees (Gardner and Gardner 1971; Terrace 1979; Terrace et al. 1979), and an orangutan (Miles 1983).

Unfortunately, claims about the signing ability of trained nonhuman primates have been met with a tide of critical literature. Among the critics are cognitive scientist Steven Pinker (1994) and linguist Noam Chomsky (1980), both of whom argue that nonhuman animals that learn to sign a handful of words are not actually engaging in linguistics but rather, at best, symbolic communication, which is fundamentally different from language because it lacks syntax and other basic structural principles, such as recursive imbedding to produce an infinite number of grammatical strings (Chomsky 1968). It has been argued that recursive thinking (i.e., the ability to think about thinking) is a central feature of human communication systems not found in other species (Hauser, Chomsky, and Fitch 2002). Clearly, one can concede that signing nonhuman primates are doing something when they sign. The question, however, is whether they are using language.

Herbert S. Terrace, the researcher who led the team that trained a chimpanzee named Nim Chimpsky (pun intended), provides further doubt that signing nonhuman primates exhibit little else than gesticulations and mimicking through operant conditioning. (Nonhuman primates are first taught to sign words by having their hands molded into signs by their trainers and then being rewarded for their successes.) Terrace reports that Nim's teachers recorded twenty thousand combinations of two or more signs over the last two years of the Nim Project, but the distributional, statistical, and semantic analyses of Nim's signing combinations were inconclusive in establishing whether Nim could construct sentences (Terrace 1979). Further damning news might be found in the fact that when Nim was relocated to live with Washoe, the first chimpanzee taught to use ASL (Gardner and Gardner 1971), neither of them attempted to communicate with the other by using signs. Both Nim and Washoe were only responsive to their trainers.

Research on the signing ability of nonhuman primates is few and far between; and disappointingly, none so far has been conducted using the requisite controls, so it is difficult to interpret the results of these projects. Nor do we have much information on chimpanzees and other nonhuman primate subjects that failed to learn any signs at all, although surely there were some who fell into this category (Candland 1993). In view of the conceptual linguistic issues raised by Pinker and Chomsky and the lack of convincing experimental evidence as admitted by Terrace, it would be premature to claim that nonhuman primates are capable of using ASL as a nonverbal language.

Controversies surrounding the definition and the enabling conditions of "beliefs" and of language notwithstanding, there may exist yet another compelling reason to suppose that the cognitive differences between humans and nonhuman primates are differences in kind. This reason comes from an emerging area in cognitive science called "embodied cognition" (Shapiro 2011). *Embodied cognition* is a general term for the view that many features of cognition are deeply dependent on the physical characteristics of a cognitive agent's body beyond the brain (Wilson and Foglia 2011). Traditionally, philosophers of mind and cognitive scientists have assumed that a cognitive agent's bodily characteristics are not directly relevant to our understanding of how cognition works. Dominant cognitive science has conceptualized cognition in terms of discrete, modular internal representations abstracted from any sensory processing and motor control. On the traditional view, cognitive functions could be accounted for locally through the genetic structures of the brain, and any physical properties beyond the brain are of interest only to the extent that they permit sensory inputs and behavioral outputs. Embodied cognition, by contrast, conceptualizes cognition as a dynamic interaction between neural and nonneural processes. For example, a cognitive agent's categorization of experienced phenomena and even spatial concepts like "up" and "down" seem to depend on the physical body of the cognitive agent (Lakoff and Johnson 1999). Beings that stand upright and walk forward may think of something's "being in front" of themselves differently from beings that are elongated and climb with gripping feet in vertical and horizontal directions (if the latter creatures have a concept of "being in front" at all). According to embodied cognition, the physical characteristics of a cognitive agent's body and how that agent interacts with its surroundings both affect the content and nature of the mental representations that it processes. Some types of cognition will come easier and some harder or not at all because of the agent's physical characteristics (think here of a dolphin's cognitive processing of its underwater environment and a human being's when similarly situated). According to this view, variations in cognition can often be attributed to variations across bodies (Wilson and Foglia 2011).[4]

If the claims of embodied cognition are true, then we might reasonably conclude that an acutely chimeric human/nonhuman primate brain in an otherwise typical nonhuman primate body would have, in virtue of just this fact alone, cognitive processes and representations that are different in kind from those of human brains in human bodies. Not even a capacious view of nonpropositional beliefs – one that would cast human and nonhuman beliefs in terms of simple imagistic mental representations – could successfully remove the substantive difference between human and nonhuman cognition, for if we take embodied cognition seriously, then humans and nonhumans would have different types of nonlinguistic "maps" or "diagrams" drawn out from their differently embodied experiences of the world.[5]

In summary, there are many controversies in cognitive science and the philosophy of mind surrounding the nature of beliefs and cognitive systems, as evidenced by just my small sample of the various positions. I pause here merely to indicate that, from this point forth in our discussion, additional theoretical controversies arise relating to other important areas. These possible disagreements are just as fundamentally important to the limit case as are the disagreements surrounding the nature of cognitive systems and beliefs.

---

[4] A concept very similar to embodied cognition, called "self-world" or *umwelt*, was espoused by Jacob von Uexküll in 1934. In the opening paragraph of his book *A Stroll through the Worlds of Animals and Men* (1934), von Uexküll asks the reader to imagine walking through a meadow strewn with insects and animals: "Here we may glimpse the worlds of the lowly dwellers of the meadow. To do so, we must first blow, in fancy, a soap bubble around each creature to represent its own world, filled with the perceptions which it alone knows.... Through the bubble we see the world of the burrowing worm, of the butterfly, or of the field mouse; the world as it appears to the animals themselves, not as it appears to us. This we may call the phenomenal world or the self-world of the animal" (von Uexküll 1934, 25).

[5] This last point might be supported further by some fascinating observations made by David and Ann Premack (1983) about the visual "maps" of chimpanzees. E.g., chimpanzees do not seem to be able to recognize two-dimensional pictures of familiar environments, such as a home or a yard that they frequent. Nor are their three-dimensional mental maps of their environments identical to ours. Premack and Premack built a replica of a chimp's room with models of furniture and objects found in the original. The chimp was able to find bait hidden in one room and transfer that information to find bait hidden in the same spot in the identical room. However, the chimp was unable to transfer bait information when the angles of one of the rooms was modified by 45 degrees. This may suggest that chimpanzees mentally map out their environments differently from humans, although this question has not been studied systematically using a statistically significant number of subjects.

Regardless of whether humans and nonhuman primates have similar or different in-kind cognitive systems, we still have to come to grips with two important guiding notions for our consideration of the limit case. In order to locate Factor X on the human side of the differences between human and nonhuman primate mental faculties, we initially have to know which mental faculties are typical for humans and which for nonhuman primates. Herein lies our next set of thorny issues. To determine the baseline of mental faculties for nonhuman primates (which we would then compare to the baseline of human mental faculties), we first have to decide what type of primates we ought to use to set our reference points. This is not simply a reminder that different nonhuman primate species may have different baselines. (In recognition of the possible variation across primate species, one would have to make sure that the baseline-setting species is the same as the host species used in the limit case.) No, the question I am posing here refers to whether we should set the baseline data by considering how nonhuman primates behave in their natural environments or whether we should use behavioral and cognitive studies conducted on nonhuman primates held in captivity and bred for research. We do not have direct access to the mental faculties of primates; thus we have to draw inferences from their observed behavior. But primates raised and held in captivity, who have never lived in a natural primate environment, behave differently from primates in the wild. Which group should set our reference standards?

Biological ethologists would argue for looking to noncaptive primates. According to them, animal behavior must be understood within the context of the animals' natural environment, not through sterile laboratory experiments that remove animals' observed behaviors from their normal social and environmental contexts (Healy and Braithwaite 2000). Ignoring the importance of these behavioral contexts could lead to a distorted view of an animal's full mental capabilities, thereby leading us to an inaccurate picture of where the baselines actually are. Consider the following analogy: marine biologists have reported that many fish and other forms of marine life lose their vibrant colors and turn gray the moment they are caught and preserved for study (Steinbeck and Ricketts 1941). Likewise, an animal's behavior may turn to a corresponding shade of "gray" in captivity and, ironically, we may lose important information about its capacities during the process of controlled study. The choice over the environmental context in which to study animals is a significant one. But in making this choice, we first have to either accept or repudiate our theoretical commitments to biological ethology.[6]

Interestingly, I believe we face a similar problem in trying to determine the baseline for human mental faculties. There is the vexing issue of exactly where to set this standard given the fact that there exists such a wide variation among human beings concerning their mental faculties, ranging from the severely developmentally challenged to the extraordinarily gifted. I wish to flag here a different problem – namely, that we are faced with another theoretical choice about ethology. Which is the best context for understanding the natural mental faculties of human beings? Are these faculties sharpest in our species during a presocial state, to which our socialization only dulls their edges, or are our faculties actualized only through our socialization? Which is the lived expression of man's true being – Tarzan or Lord Greystoke? The eighteenth-century philosopher Jean-Jacques Rousseau would argue on behalf of Tarzan. Rousseau believed that the genuine qualities of human beings can only be understood when the distorting influences of society are removed. He lamented, however, that this self-understanding could not be achieved in his time:

> [H]ow will man manage to see himself as nature formed him, through all the changes that the sequence of time and things must have produced in his original constitution, and to separate what he gets from his own stock from what circumstances and his progress have added to or changed in his primitive state? Like the statue of Glaucus, which time, sea, and storms had so disfigured that it looked less like a god than a wild beast, the human soul, altered in the bosom of society by a thousand continually renewed causes, by the acquisition of a mass of knowledge and errors, by changes that occurred in the constitution of bodies, and by the continual impact of the passions, has, so to speak, changed its appearance to the point of being nearly unrecognizable.... (1754, 91)

One may object that, even if we accept Rousseau's idealized view of our long-lost "original constitution," this view does us no good for the limit

---

[6] This debate about ethology can be traced back as far as the late 1800s, early 1900s. Richard L. Garner (1896) argued that ape behavior should be studied in the wild, while Lightner Witmer (1909) countered that the mental abilities of apes should be studied under controlled laboratory conditions. Both tried to teach chimpanzees to speak under these respective (opposite) conditions; both failed. Edward L. Thorndike (1898), one of the founders of behaviorism, believed that the mental abilities of animals could be studied systematically and devised the now-famous "puzzle box" to measure the learning rates of cats, dogs, and chickens. From these studies we get the concept of the learning curve (or as Thorndike called it, a "time curve"). T. Wesley Mills (1898), a vocal critic of Thorndike, argued that an animal uncomfortable with its environment will reveal none of its true abilities.

case, because, according to even Rousseau, man's unsocialized original state of being cannot be known by us. However, I believe we must not be so dismissive of Rousseau's point, for if he is right that the current state of human faculties is the product of vastly accumulated social influences, then it may be unfair and distorting to compare the raw, emergent mental faculties of acute neurological chimeras to the socially cultivated faculties of modern man. Human/nonhuman acute neurological chimeras in our limit case would be born into laboratory conditions more closely approximating a presocial and primitive state rather than an environment that would further shape their mental faculties within the "bosom of society." Postnatal neurological chimeras are not likely to undergo the kind of interaction and socialization that human newborns receive from the day they are brought home to the family network. Instead, they are much more likely to be studied under sterile laboratory conditions and housed under (less-than-human) requirements of environmental enrichment deemed appropriate for the host nonhuman primate species. To dismiss Rousseau's point as irrelevant to our limit case is to assume that Tarzan's faculties can be appropriately measured against to those of an English aristocrat, and that undistorted and unbiased conclusions can be drawn from this comparison regarding the limits of Tarzan's faculties.

Our dilemma then is this. The fairest way to compare the mental faculties of neurological chimeras and human beings would be to compare the faculties of the former to the faculties of man in a comparably asocial and primitive state. But the conditions of the latter are not known by us.[7] The alternative would be to compare the mental faculties of chimeras with the mental faculties of socially developed human beings. But then this would first have to involve, for the sake of comparative equity, the fulfillment of a comparable offer of social development for chimeric nonhuman primates. The first alternative may not be achievable. The

---

[7] One might propose that our limited knowledge of feral children may help us set the baseline for asocial man, but I believe this is a poor solution. We would have to run the same behavioral and cognitive tests on the neurological chimera group and on feral children, and we simply do not have the latter to fulfill the role of the control group, nor can we produce feral children for this purpose for obvious ethical reasons. Furthermore, using the few existing published accounts of feral children is problematic as a type of "historical control group." Some have speculated that feral children were abandoned by their parents due to their having a congenital mental handicap, and other feral children were known to have experienced extreme abuse (torture and years of solitary confinement) that may have offsetting effects on the expression of their innate mental faculties. See Douglas Candland's excellent overview of feral children (1993). Notably, no feral children ever learned to use language (most would frequently slip into a catatonic state), and one of them reportedly did not recognize his own reflection in a mirror.

second alternative is not impossible, but it is highly unlikely to be carried out on neurological chimeras that have been brought into existence for the sake of invasive stem cell–based research, not behavioral studies aimed at assessing their mental faculties related to moral status.

So here we stand, limited in our progress toward evaluating the limit case due to the uncertainties surrounding the nature of cognitive systems, the nature of beliefs, the implications of embodied cognition, and the appropriate baseline-setting reference classes for human and non-human primate cognitive agents. Is there a way to proceed in our consideration of the limit case without decisively settling any one of these complex philosophical issues?

## Self-Consciousness

Some may argue that there is. Some may argue that we should look to *self-consciousness* as an appropriate candidate for Factor X. This seems to be a reasonable choice. Self-consciousness appears to fulfill the two main desiderata for Factor X: it is a human mental faculty that nonhuman primates seem to lack (or at least, as I discuss in the following text, it may be doubted that they do) and it is morally important. Let us suppose for the sake of argument then that we identify Factor X with self-consciousness without first making any theoretical commitments on the issues previously discussed. How far can we get using this strategy?

It appears not very far. Self-consciousness can be roughly defined as a cognitive agent's ability to recognize itself as having mental experiences. This rough definition needs further clarification. For one, self-consciousness should not be confused with consciousness in the sense of one's being wakeful or alert (as opposed to one's being anesthetized or in a coma). We can concede that nonhuman primates and other animals are conscious in this latter sense. Furthermore, the notion of self-consciousness we are after should be distinguished from other notions that might get included under this label. Sometimes people use the term *self-consciousness* to mean simple self-discernment. But there are important differences between these notions (Allen and Bekoff 1997). Simple self-discernment occurs in many nonhuman animals, and for this reason alone it is a poor candidate for Factor X in our limit case. Clearly nonhuman animals are self-discerning in the sense that they are able to distinguish themselves from their offspring, pack mates, or other flocking birds during coordinated flight. And certainly nonhuman animals can distinguish the real movements of objects in their sensory fields from apparent movements produced by their own motions (Barresi and Moore 1996). However, none of these examples of simple self-discernment necessitates that nonhuman animals must be aware that they are making these distinctions. The concept of self-consciousness we are after here is more complex than simple self-discernment. Hereafter, by *self-consciousness* I shall mean a kind of higher-level self-awareness that comes from thinking about thinking (or what some have called recursive thinking). To be self-conscious in this sense, a being must have a higher-order mental awareness of its own mental states (Allen 2010).

Self-consciousness in this more robust sense is closely related to what philosophers and cognitive scientists call theory of mind. The term *theory of mind* was introduced by David Premack and Guy Woodruff (1978), who defined it as one's ability to predict and explain behavior by attributing mental states to others. (For illustrative purposes, think here of a magician distracting his audience with one hand while producing a trick with the other. Magicians practice their trade by producing and playing upon their audience's false beliefs, which would be impossible if either the magician or his audience lacked a theory of mind.) Theory of mind and self-consciousness are related in that the former is a by-product of the latter; one realizes, self-consciously, that one is a minded being, and one presumes that others are similarly minded (Gallup et al. 2002).

Both self-consciousness and its offshoot, theory of mind, are morally important mental characteristics. Without self-consciousness an individual could not be an autonomous moral agent, let alone a being that could take a reflective interest in its own continued existence.[8] Furthermore, without a theory of mind, a being could not draw a distinction between its own mental states and others' mental states, let alone attribute beliefs and desires to individuals to predict their actions. I dare venture to say that the very possibility of secular ethics depends on the existence of beings that are self-conscious and have a theory of mind.

Having made these distinctions, the key questions for us to consider then are, do nonhuman primates have self-consciousness and, if not, is self-consciousness something that can be gained through acute human/ nonhuman chimerization? In attempting to address these questions, we find our earlier philosophical concerns forcing themselves back into our

---

[8] I believe it is this capacity for self-consciousness that philosophers like Frankfurt (1971) implicitly use to ground their hierarchical conceptions of individual autonomy. Frankfurt argues that an individual is a person in virtue of his or her capacity to form second-order volitions (i.e., higher-order desires to have one's particular first-order desire move one to act). See my discussion of autonomy in the respect for persons section of Chapter 3.

consideration, especially questions surrounding the nature of beliefs and the importance of biological ethology. If self-consciousness involves the capacity to have second-order mental representations of one's own mental states, then self-consciousness must involve propositionally grounded beliefs, not solely beliefs that are cashed out in terms of nonpropositional, first-order mental representations (mental pictures or maps). If this is true, then nonhuman primates cannot have self-consciousness, at least not without propositional beliefs and the ability to think recursively, both of which are intimately tied to language use.

Critics may object that some experimental evidence has shown that nonhuman primates (mainly chimpanzees) can have self-consciousness and a theory of mind, despite their lack of language. For example, in 1970 Gordon Gallup pioneered the "mirror test," which has been widely followed as a protocol for testing the presence of self-consciousness in animals. In his seminal study, Gallup anesthetized chimpanzee subjects and marked their foreheads with a dye (the control group was anesthetized only). Upon waking, the chimpanzees were shown a mirror. The marked chimpanzees touched their foreheads more frequently than the control chimpanzees, suggesting that chimpanzees can recognize themselves in mirror images (Gallup 1970).

People have taken results such as these as proof that chimpanzees are self-conscious. However it should be noted out that of the 163 chimpanzees tested across the scientific literature, only 73 "passed" the mirror test (Shumaker and Swartz 2002). Evidence of mirror self-recognition in primate species outside of the great apes is even sparser. Do these results prove that chimpanzees and other great apes have self-consciousness?

There are reasons for people on both sides of the issue to be skeptical of what may be concluded from mirror test studies.[9] Those who doubt the existence of self-consciousness in nonhuman primates are not impressed by the percentage of subjects who have "passed" the mirror test. Furthermore, doubters may question whether mark-touching behavior is a reliable indicator of an animal subject's interest in *itself* (using the image as a proxy for its own self) and not an interest simply in the image reflected in the mirror (Allen 2010). Believers of nonhuman primate

---

[9] Personally, I find the mirror test to be a highly anthropomorphic conceit. The notion of looking at oneself in a mirror and noticing a mark on one's forehead seems to signify a great deal more about how humans typically use mirrors than how nonhuman primates might express an awareness of self, which may be, for all we know, cued in some nonvisual way. The mirror test may simply be irrelevant as a test for self-consciousness in nonhumans.

self-consciousness, by contrast, may be wary of whether the mirror test is ethologically valid, because nonhuman primates do not look at their reflections in the wild and some subjects may have to learn to become accustomed to making direct eye contact. Gorillas are averse to making direct eye contact, and this may help explain why mirror test results are so dismal for this species, with only six out of twenty-three subjects exhibiting mark-touching behavior (Shumaker and Swartz 2002).

It is also uncertain, if not even more doubtful, that nonhuman primates have a theory of mind. Recall that theory of mind is a derivative of self-consciousness, so if one lacks self-consciousness, then one cannot have a theory of mind. Nonverbal tests used to assess the presence of theory of mind in primates have not shown that they understand the notion of a false belief (Call and Tomasello 2008). For example, chimpanzee subjects in one study were shown their competitors being deceived about the location of food, but they did not use this tip to their own advantage, suggesting that they did not understand that their competitors had been misled (Kaminski et al. 2008).

In light of the current scientific evidence, it does not appear that believers have established that nonhuman primates have self-consciousness or a theory of mind. This lack of strong empirical evidence should be added to our previously mentioned philosophical point that self-consciousness involves second-order mental representations that are difficult to conceive of as anything other than recursively embedded propositional beliefs. In my opinion, the net sum of these empirical and philosophical considerations should lead one to conclude that nonhuman primates do not have self-consciousness (although they are certainly sentient, highly intelligent, and capable of simple self-discernment). Admittedly, the absence of evidence does not logically entail evidence of absence (Allen 2010), but the burden of proof lies with those who insist on something's actually being the case, such as the claim that nonhuman primates have self-consciousness. And thus far, behavioral research on nonhuman primates has not been terribly convincing on this score.

Perhaps part of others' and my reluctance to accept whether nonhuman primates have self-consciousness may be attributable to the fact that, as a matter of empirical methodologically, we must draw our conclusions inferentially for nonhuman primate behavioral studies. The problem is that different reasonable people can infer different conclusions using the same data. For the purposes of our discussion, there are two ways to argue for the presence of self-consciousness (or any other human mental faculty) in nonhuman primates. One is an argument from analogy: (1) we suppose human beings are self-conscious; (2) human beings exhibit certain behaviors in virtue of being self-conscious; (3) nonhuman primates exhibit one or more of these same types of behavior; (4) therefore, nonhuman primates have self-consciousness. Another argument is what is called inference to the best explanation: (1) nonhuman primates exhibit a certain type of behavior; (2) the best explanation for their engaging in this behavior is that they have self-consciousness; (3) therefore, nonhuman primates are self-conscious. Both of these inferential methods of argument are open to attack. Arguments from analogy are vulnerable to doubts as to whether the apparent similarities between two groups entail that both groups share the same underlying cause for their similarities. Doubters can also exploit the presence of dissimilarities between groups to undermine analogy arguments. Arguments based on inference to the best explanation are plagued by doubts as to whether we have hit upon the best scientific explanation for an observed phenomenon or whether we are simply limited in our own scientific and theoretical imaginations and have not fully considered other possible explanations.

In addition to these problems, inferential reasoning about nonhuman primate self-consciousness may also be susceptible to various degrees of anthropomorphism. In Chapter 5, I discussed people's propensity to slip into old folk beliefs in the face of uncertainty, beliefs that would attribute to nonhuman animals some very human traits. Many animal behavior researchers may be just as liable to slip unconsciously into this familiar pattern. This is not a criticism, just a conjecture. People for whom the lives of animals matter very deeply may feel that discovering differences between humans and animals is far less joyful than finding similarities. The "killjoy" quality of discovering differences may motivate observers to find more similarities in the face of ambiguous data (Andrews 2011; Shettleworth 2010). As an animal lover I can certainly appreciate this tendency to attribute humanlike psychological states, motivations, and emotions to the animals I value. But perhaps this says much more about the kind of person I am than the kind of beings my companion animals are. Anthropomorphism may simply be our theory of mind gone overboard, whereby we attribute self-consciousness and other human mental traits to animals without adequate justification.

In the absence of convincing evidence to the contrary, I propose that human beings are different from nonhuman primates in the sense that humans typically have the mental faculty of self-consciousness. If this is true, then we may have found our Factor X. Whatever else human beings are cognitively capable of doing, their having self-consciousness seems sufficient to fulfill the determinative role we have been seeking in our chimera limit case. Rather than searching for the presence of an array of various human cognitive capacities in chimeric animals, we can limit our search to this one key factor. Self-consciousness nicely encapsulates other aspects of human cognition that many philosophers and cognitive scientists would argue are unique to human beings. Having self-consciousness requires propositional beliefs and recursive thinking, both of which have a supportive role in other important human capabilities, such as language use, theory of mind, romantic love, the arts, and so forth.

It should be noted that in identifying Factor X with self-consciousness, I am taking a stand on many of the philosophical issues outlined in this chapter. Most importantly, I am claiming that the differences between human cognitive systems and animal cognitive systems are differences in kind. This is a judgment I am happy to live with, for I believe alternative positions that attempt to eliminate any metaphysical difference between human beliefs and "animal beliefs" come at too high of a philosophical cost. Lost would be the intuitively appealing notion that, when I introspect on my own beliefs, I find that my beliefs are clearly propositional – that they are mental representations of the world and of concepts that I know can be true or false, consistent or inconsistent. (Truth and falsity, consistency and inconsistency are properties only of propositions.) The same sort of simple introspection about the nature of one's own beliefs is not possible for nonhuman primates because they need propositions to have such second-order beliefs. To rate human beliefs as similar in kind to nonhuman primate beliefs impoverishes the notion of human belief. It is difficult for me to imagine how anyone could possibly entertain philosophical questions such as the ones I have been posing in this chapter if it were not for the fact that human beliefs are propositional.

The preceding discussions are not meant to be merely philosophical and academic; they have real implications for how we oversee stem cell–based chimera research at the practical research ethics level. If the emergence of self-consciousness is a decisive factor in our judgment of the moral status of human/nonhuman neurological chimeras, then we must employ empirical tests to assess whether self-consciousness is present in a chimeric research subject. How one is supposed to devise such a test is a mystery to me, especially for beings that lack language. The mirror test discussed in the preceding text seems inadequate, because it is difficult to know what mark-touching behavior is supposed to signify about the presence of self-consciousness (understood here as a subject's having second-order mental representations of its own mental states). Neither could we straightforwardly use a false belief test to indicate that neurological chimeras have a theory of mind (and therefore also self-consciousness). Human children are unable to pass false belief tests prior to the age of four (Wimmer and Perner 1983), and yet none of us would deny that children eventually arrive at having a theory of mind. This developmental fact suggests we would similarly have to raise acute neurological chimeras to a comparable point of maturity before expecting any of them to be even remotely capable of passing a false belief test. Admittedly, none of this amounts to a proof that it would be impossible to devise a self-consciousness test (or, by proxy, a theory of mind test) for acute neurological chimeras. But even if such tests were created, we still have to be prepared to face the fact that the results of any self-consciousness test for language-less chimeras are liable to be questioned by doubters of inferential argumentation.

## Some Preliminary Conclusions

I began this chapter with what is perhaps the most highly charged issue surrounding stem cell–based chimera research – acute neurological chimerism of nonhuman primates using human stem cells or their direct derivatives. Many people may be deeply concerned about what might happen to the moral status of the research animal if such extreme biological blending were to occur. However, to have the thought that the acute neurological chimerism of nonhuman primates might lead to their moral humanization is to leave that thought unfinished. To finish the thought, we need to take seriously the range of philosophical issues that I have raised in this chapter and we need to take a stance on many of these theoretical controversies. Our consideration of the limit case reveals a series of competing claims for which one must first choose one divergent side or another before anything interesting can be said about the ethics of the limit case. These competing claims involve the nature of cognitive systems and beliefs, the implications of embodied cognition and biological ethology, and the proper baseline-setting reference classes for human and nonhuman primate cognitive agents. Depending on the positions one takes on these background issues, one will conclude (with varying degrees of personal conviction) that acute neurological chimerism is or is not likely to transform nonhuman primate hosts into beings that possess full moral status. I leave it up to the reader to decide which of these conclusions he or she finds more plausible.

For my part, I have taken a stance on these background issues. As a result of my own theoretical commitments, I have suggested that self-consciousness (understood here as one's higher-order mental awareness of one's own mental states) is the right mental faculty to serve the role of Factor X in our limit case. Self-consciousness requires the cognitive agent to have recursive, propositionally grounded beliefs tied to language use. As such, self-consciousness meets the main requirements we were searching for in Factor X – it is a morally important mental trait present in humans but not nonhuman primates. As such, self-consciousness is not likely to emerge in nonhuman primate neurological chimeras, for its emergence would necessitate a very dramatic and categorical shift in the typical cognitive system of the host species. That is, a human/nonhuman chimeric brain would have to begin organizing its mental representations using propositionally grounded beliefs and generate metabeliefs about these first-order beliefs. But not even brains that are 100 percent biologically human are always guaranteed to produce self-consciousness in this sense.

Furthermore, I have highlighted the challenges involved in devising a test for self-consciousness for neurologically chimeric nonhuman primates that lack language. In these situations, the best we can do is employ empirical procedures to support inferential conclusions using arguments from analogy or inference to the best explanation. Both of these argumentative strategies, however, are open to doubt by skeptics of nonhuman self-consciousness.

Added to these logical limitations is a formidable practical constraint. Self-consciousness is a complex mental faculty that takes years to emerge, as our common experience with human infants indicates. Assuming the same kind of developmental fact applies to neurological chimeras, these nonhuman subjects would have to be housed and nurtured under humanlike socialization processes within the "bosom of society" before we can hope to see any signs of self-consciousness. Unfortunately, serious attempts to situate neurological chimeras in a position favorable for revealing any chimerically generated capacity for self-consciousness are likely to be extremely time and labor intensive and, perhaps most importantly, in deep conflict with the invasive experimental purposes for which stem cell–based neurological chimeras would be created and maintained in laboratories in the first place. It should be noted that extensive socialization and language acquisition efforts in the past involving nonhuman (unchimerized) primates produced no evidence of humanlike self-consciousness; so there seems to be little reason to expect drastically different outcomes with neuro-logical chimeras.[10]

## What Else Might the Limit Case Teach Us?

The issues I have raised in this chapter are rich and complex. Together, they would be well served by a book-length treatment in their own right. I reluctantly draw my discussion to a close with these last few observations.

Some readers may grow impatient with the theoretical haze that has gathered around the limit case. Some may be tempted to toss out the philosophical questions I have raised in this chapter and focus instead on developing and refining the self-consciousness and theory of mind tests that have already been employed on nonhuman primates. However, pushing ahead in this practically minded manner would be a grave mistake.

I believe there is a sense in which the central questions we have discussed in this chapter are scientifically intractable, or at least a sense in which they resist clear empirical solutions. This problem is more fundamental than the logical weaknesses associated with arguments from analogy and inference to the best explanation (which remain, as I have noted several times, vulnerable to doubt). The deeper problem here can be stated as follows: we need to know what we are looking for when assessing neurological chimeras for the emergence of "important human qualities" – qualities that would make the continuation of a chimera research protocol unethical, that is, what I have called Factor X. Any test for the presence of Factor X must be devised first in light of the particular conception of Factor X that the test was designed to pick out; as a result, the test cannot be used to vindicate or rationalize one's starting notion of Factor X.[11] If one believes that Factor X is self-consciousness,

---

[10] A few chimpanzees were raised for years in the same manner as human infants by researchers who hoped to narrow their cognitive gap to human beings. These lengthy socialization experiments produced no significant results (Candland 1993; Hayes 1951; Kellogg and Kellogg 1933).

[11] The philosophical error in reversing this order is nicely illustrated by the following example. Imagine that your friend is walking around town carrying a bizarre telescopic viewing device that he has made. You ask him what this device is. He says, "This is my WHAT'S-IT finder – I use it to find WHAT'S-ITs." "What's a WHAT'S-IT?" you ask him. He replies, "Whatever I find using this finder." The philosophical joke here is that one first needs to know what a WHAT'S-IT is before one builds a WHAT'S-IT finder. Otherwise the design of the finder is arbitrary. I owe this example to Marc Alspector-Kelly.

then one cannot simply take a shortcut to the empirical methods for detecting it and skip the philosophical analyses necessary to clarify our ideas about what self-consciousness is and what its basic enabling conditions are. Thus we have no alternative but to wade first through the theoretical haze.

Prior to our sustained exploration of the limit case in this chapter, I believe it was quite easy to overstate the threat of moral humanization in chimeric animals. Without expending the mental energy necessary to analyze exactly what moral humanization would need to involve, people's thoughts were liable to fly toward fancies of what it is possible to imagine. But if we expose the chain of easy assumptions that are leapfrogged on these flights of the imagination, then perhaps people's anxieties surrounding the limit case might be assuaged to some extent. I have suggested that, from a philosophical standpoint, the moral humanization of neurological chimeras is not some imminent threat just waiting to be triggered by a stem cell experiment.

However, I admit that the type of analysis I have offered in this chapter may work on an intellectual level for many, but it might not succeed in dislodging people's deep-seated fears. As I discussed in Chapter 5, there are attitudes and tendencies toward mythological thinking that seem to be part of the very structure of the human psyche. If this supposition is true, then people's concerns about chimera research and their fears surrounding the limit case may speak volumes more about themselves than the real-life possibilities they profess to be describing. When boundaries cross, when binaries appear to come into direct opposition, how people respond to these perceptions, how they come to reconcile these contradictions in their own minds may reveal little more than their own uncertainties about the human condition. Again, John Steinbeck and Ed Ricketts expressed this point most beautifully when they wrote:

> Man might be described fairly adequately, if simply, as a two-legged paradox. He has never become accustomed to the tragic miracle of consciousness. Perhaps, as has been suggested, his species is not set, has not jelled, but is still in a state of becoming, bound by his physical memories of a past of struggle and survival, limited in his futures by the uneasiness of thought and consciousness. (Steinbeck and Ricketts 1941, 96)

It appears to me that it is man's "uneasiness of thought and consciousness" that is under siege in the debate over neurological chimera research, so it should come as little surprise if people's anxieties in this area prove to be the most difficult to mollify through reasoned, philosophical debate.

## Conclusion

It is apparent to me that the acute neurological chimerism of nonhuman primates is truly the limit case in the fullest sense of the term. We are limited in several ways: in what we know about the biological effects of transferring large quantities of human neural matter into developing nonhuman primate brains; in knowing what goes on in the silent minds of nonhuman primates; (thankfully) in many regions of the world in what we may do to nonhuman primates for research purposes, particularly the great apes; and in what we can say about the possibility for moral humanization without further philosophical thought on the theoretical and practical matters I have raised in this chapter.

Given my own theoretical commitments, I am not personally worried about the chances that acute neurological chimerism could produce self-consciousness in nonhuman primate hosts, for such biological blending would have to amount to a truly astonishing and radical transformation in their cognitive systems. Chimeric brains would have to function at least as well as wholly human brains in their ability to support a metaawareness of propositionally grounded mental representations of the world, all without the aid of language. Although I have no proof that this is impossible, I am highly doubtful it is likely, especially given the further, socially based developmental rearing requirements necessary to support any such latent ability. In view of these preliminary conclusions concerning the limit case, some observers may reason that our ethical concerns about the possibility of moral humanization ought to drop off sharply when it comes to research animals outside the primate species and far below the limit-case level. This, I hope, will be the minimal effect of my preceding discussions.

Some observers who are less confident about their conclusions may wonder whether the shroud of uncertainty surrounding the limit case could justify for many researchers an "anything goes" approach to acute neurological chimera research with nonhuman primates. Hardly. At the beginning of this chapter I deliberately focused our attention on the philosophical issues by conveniently setting aside some important real-world issues and constraints pertaining to the limit case. We ought to bring these practical considerations back into our discussion now. Readers will recall that among the ethical requirements for animal research are that there is no other way to answer the research question and there are no other animal species with a greater evolutionary distance from us that can serve as appropriate hosts for the chimera study. I believe that, on a case-by-case basis, serious doubts can be raised as to whether stem cell investigators can mount a convincing argument that these preconditions have been met to justify their use of nonhuman primates. Added to this is a notable skepticism among many scientists that the developmental interactions between the derived human neural cells and the host primate's would not be very indicative of what would happen in a fully human biological context. We may never know how human stem cell products will behave in a human body until we transfer them into human research subjects in a clinical trial. Human stem cell–based clinical trials and their accompanying ethical difficulties is the topic Chapter 7.

In conclusion, I believe people's attention should remain squarely on the issue of animal welfare, as discussed in Chapter 5. Unlike moral humanization, animal suffering and acute biological dysfunction are the far more present and likely effects of neurological chimerism. It is perhaps an extreme form of arrogance – an unstated moral imperialism connected to human stem cells – to assume that the transfer of human neural matter into nonhuman brains will end up enhancing research animals above their typical species functioning. The more likely result, if our past experience with transgenic animals is a guide, would be a precipitous drop in animal welfare. This is why the ISSCR Ethics and Public Policy Committee focused its attention on drafting chimera research guidelines that placed animal welfare at the top of its list of regulatory priorities. If one opposes the use of nonhuman primates in stem cell–based chimera research, one should oppose it on grounds other than the moral humanization concern, for animal welfare issues are much more real, probable, and tractable through empirical methods for assessing pain and suffering. The true heuristic value of the limit case, I believe, just might lie in our coming to this more level-headed conclusion.

# 7

## Human Trials

### *Testing Stem Cell–Based Biologics in Patients*

A trial may be broadly defined as an organized process of testing or examination to determine whether something is or is not the case, be it a person's guilt or innocence (criminal trials), an athlete's qualification for competition (time trials), a ship's seaworthiness (sea trials), a medical intervention's safety and efficacy (clinical trials), and so forth. Presumably, the outcome of a trial is unknown from the start. Hence the need to have a go at an assessment (the term *trial* comes from the Anglo-French *trier* – to try). At the beginning of a trial there is uncertainty. At the end, it is hoped there will be less uncertainty. Any marginal gain in assurance is dependent on the reliability and objectivity of the trial in question.

Each of these points is plainly obvious to anyone who entertains the general notion of a trial. To these simple observations I add a few more in this introductory section. Together, these commonly held understandings provide us with an initial framework for thinking about the ethics of stem cell–based clinical trials, which is the focus of this chapter.

All trials can be viewed from multiple perspectives. First, there is the point of view of the individual or individuals undergoing the trial, the outcome of which is determinative of some important personal interest. Second, there is the point of view of those administering the trial, the process of which is their responsibility to administer accurately and fairly. Third, there is the point of view of other parties distinct from the first two – namely, third parties who may have some further interest in the outcome of the trial, be that economic, emotional, or social interest, and so forth. Trials typically have a conventionally agreed upon endpoint, or at least a set of stopping rules, at which time the matter under examination can be assessed relative to each party's interests. Finally, trials are conducted in reference to some recognized standard for evaluation. In

summary these commonplace observations are applicable to any type of
trial, be it for sport, justice, engineering, or medical advancements: (1)
trials test matters of uncertainty, (2) trials must be reliable and objective,
(3) different parties can have varying interests regarding a trial's outcome,
(4) trials have either an agreed upon endpoint or clear stopping rules,
and (5) trials presuppose the existence of some recognized standard.
That said, it is surprising the degree to which these common stipulations
get confounded when it comes to stem cell–based clinical trials.

### Different Perspectives, Different Interests

In order best to appreciate the ethical, scientific, and regulatory complexities surrounding stem cell–based clinical trials, it is worth first
acknowledging the multiple perspectives and interests at play, beginning
with the point of view of the patient.

A Parkinson's disease patient once described to me his illness as a kind
of "trial by ordeal."[1] This, I believe, is a beautiful metaphor, not only
for conveying many patients' personal struggles with their intractable
diseases, but also for depicting their hopes in volunteering for a clinical trial. Historically, a trial by ordeal was a medieval juridical method
of determining a person's guilt or innocence by subjecting the accused
to a dangerous task believed to be under divine control (Bartlett 1986).
The accused were considered innocent if they survived the test or if their
injuries healed. Trials by water and trials by fire were among the most
common forms of trial by ordeal (Figure 7.1).

Faith was an essential element of these early juridical tests, for the
premoderns believed that God would intervene to help the innocent
endure their trials by ordeal. Similarly, many religious patients today
seem to cope with their intractable diseases by believing that their experiences are a test of faith. Although perhaps not always praying for a cure,
many patients may see their illnesses as an opportunity to strengthen
their bonds with God and others.[2] In this way, intractable diseases could
be regarded by some as a trial by ordeal, not of guilt or innocence, but
of faith and inner strength. On this view, God can help patients endure
their trial by ordeal if they submit themselves to Him.

[1] I owe this metaphor to Tom Isaacs, a Parkinson's disease patient and the cofounder of
The Cure Parkinson's Trust, United Kingdom.
[2] Perhaps one of the most famous patients who maintained this sort of belief was Pope
John Paul II, who was afflicted with symptomatic Parkinson's disease during the last
twelve years of his life (Weigel 2005).

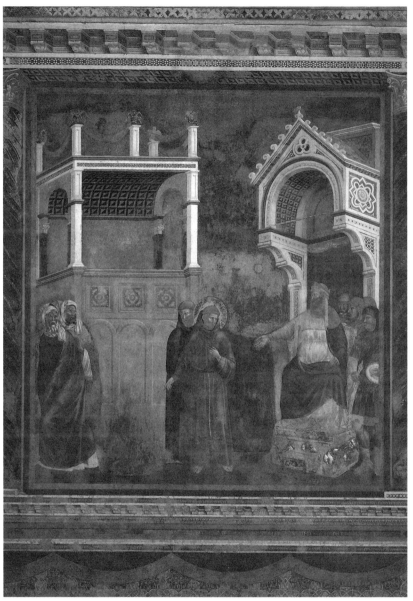

FIGURE 7.1. Saint Francis undergoing the trial by fire.
Credit: Scala/Art Resource, NY. Description: Scenes from the Life of
Saint Francis: The Ordeal by Fire. Artist: Giotto di Bondone (1266–1336).
Location: S. Francesco, Assisi, Italy.

The trial by ordeal metaphor is also an apt symbol for portraying some patients' motivations for enrolling in a clinical trial. By submitting themselves to a clinical trial, some patients may hope to be cured – or at least therapeutically improved – in the process. Here, the patient's trial by ordeal is embodied through a clinical study in which medical science, either acting alone or as an agent of God's will, might enable the sick to fight against their disease.[3] On this view, patients put their faith in medical science.

Both these interpretations of the trial by ordeal metaphor offer important insights. The first interpretation reminds us that chronic, intractable diseases can be a deeply personal experience and that many patients face not only an intense physical crisis but a spiritual one as well. The second interpretation reminds us that some patients may enroll in a clinical trial under the motive of a therapeutic misconception or, if not on the basis of a factual error, then at least under the drive of a therapeutic hope for themselves or for other patients like them.[4] Hope and faith are the common threads that unite the two interpretations of the trial by ordeal metaphor. If we want to understand stem cell–based clinical trials and the disease experience from the patient's point of view, we must remind ourselves that the patient's vantage point is very often filtered through the lens of faith and hope.[5]

[3]  Timothy Atchinson, the first patient to receive embryonic stem cell–derived oligodendrocytes in a spinal cord–injury clinical trial, is quoted in the *Washington Post* as saying that his injury and his involvement in Geron's stem cell clinical trial are part of God's will (Stein 2011).

[4]  The fifth, and final, patient to be enrolled in Geron's spinal cord–injury trial, Katie Sharify, is quoted in the *San Francisco Chronicle* as saying that she decided to participate in the clinical trial because she hoped her involvement could help a patient like herself in the future (Allday 2011). She says, "I'd been trying to find a reason all of this happened to me." Ms. Sharify had embryonic stem cell–derived oligodendrocytes injected into her injured spinal cord just two days after Geron announced it was abandoning its stem cell research division and ending its clinical trial. I discuss the Geron trial later in this chapter.

[5]  It goes without saying that hope and faith are concepts that have rich and complex religious histories. E.g., according to Paul the Apostle in 1 Corinthians 13:13, hope and faith are identified as two of the main elements of Christian character, alongside love (*agape*) (Easton 1897). Meanwhile, Islam instructs Muslims to regard faith as a dedication to certain behaviors and deeds, most notably the five pillars of Islam: confession of faith, prayer five times daily, alms, fasting in the month of Ramadan, and pilgrimage to Mecca (Nasr 2002).

Regardless of whether one is of a religious persuasion, it is important to note here that hope, like its cousin faith, is a concept that need not conform to modern standards of rationality and thus cannot be easily criticized or dismissed simply for failing to meet modernist rational norms.

Much has been written about the therapeutic misconception in human subjects research. The notion of therapeutic misconception has traditionally been understood in the bioethics and medical literature as a research subject's false belief that "every aspect of the research project to which he had consented was designed to benefit him directly" (Appelbaum et al. 1987, 20). Subjects who operate under this false belief do so in part because they do not adequately understand randomization or double blinding in scientific research. And even when subjects do cognitively grasp these concepts, they usually have a hard time genuinely believing that researchers would not necessarily be acting in their best interests and that there could be any major disadvantages to participating in the research (Appelbaum et al. 1982). As a result, many research subjects may mistakenly believe that they are consenting to interventions designed to treat their illness rather than to produce generalizable scientific knowledge. For example, in a recent study of cancer patients enrolled in an early phase clinical trial, the vast majority were reported to confuse exploratory biomedical research with actual treatment and had difficulty understanding the differences between the two (Pentz et al. 2012). In essence, therapeutic misconception is a matter of having inaccurate information and beliefs, the presence of which undermine the autonomy of a patient's choice to consent to research participation.

Therapeutic hope, by contrast, is not the same as therapeutic misconception, and we must not confuse the two. Unfortunately, it is a notion that has received far less attention than therapeutic misconception (Hyun 2006a). Some patient subjects might be motivated to participate in stem cell–based clinical trials, not by false beliefs about the exploratory nature of this research, but by hopes for what the research could yield for themselves or their loved ones. In these cases, the concept of a therapeutic misconception may not provide the best tool for ethical analysis. Therapeutic hope can exist in cases in which there is a very slim chance that volunteering for a particular medical research could lead to physical improvements for the patient, even if the study is not actually designed to produce health benefits for the research subject. In these situations, it is not so easy to talk patients out of participating in research, particularly if it is not certain that the study intervention would have zero chance of improving the patient's condition. Therapeutic hope survives wherever there exists even the most remote chance of benefit.[6] I shall

---

[6] A parallel point has been made in the bioethics literature concerning the notion of medical futility. As long as it is not physically impossible for a medical intervention to have an

return to this issue in Chapter 8, but for now I simply wish to flag the concern that therapeutic hope, like therapeutic misconception, is ethically problematic because it can leave the patient subject vulnerable to exploitation. The cure for therapeutic misconception is to correct the patient's false beliefs. The cure for therapeutic hope, if a cure for this is desirable, is not so obvious.

Besides the patient's point of view – that is, the point of view of the individual involved as a research subject in a stem cell–based clinical trial – there is also the vantage point of others not directly undergoing a clinical trial, but who may have some other interest in its outcome nonetheless. (These other individuals are symbolized by the crowd surrounding Saint Francis standing at the center of Figure 7.1.) In its most generalized sense this outsider's perspective could be identified as the vantage point of society at large. But we must be careful not to assume that the societal point of view is one homogenous unit, for society is comprised, in part, by proponents and opponents of embryonic stem cell research, each of whom might track the progress of early stage stem cell–based clinical trials to vindicate their own political opinions about the moral permissibility of embryo-derived stem cell research.

At the time of this writing, minor successes and worrying setbacks have been reported for early stage embryonic stem cell–derived clinical studies. Researchers from UCLA and the stem cell biotech company Advanced Cell Technology (ACT) announced their mutual work on two prospective clinical studies to establish the safety and tolerability of using hES cell–derived cells to treat two similar forms of blindness. Researchers transplanted hES cell–derived retinal pigment epithelium into the eyes of two patients, one suffering from Stargardt's macular dystrophy and the other from dry age-related macular degeneration. Both of these prospective clinical studies produced encouraging data four months posttransplant (Schwartz et al. 2012). For example, neither of the patients described in this report experienced additional vision loss, nor was there any evidence of cell hyperproliferation, tumors, or immune rejection. And both of these patients gained minor improvements in their visual acuity. As a result of this preliminary report, ACT was given approval to enroll additional patients in their stem cell–based study. In contrast to these incremental successes, the world's first embryonic stem cell–derived spinal cord–injury trial was halted by its sponsor

effect desired by the patient or his or her family, then it is a mistake for others to dismiss a desire for this intervention as simply irrational. In these cases, the desire to attempt a medical intervention with a very low probability for success is fueled by hope and a value-driven commitment to at least give that intervention a try (Youngner 1988).

Geron after it was announced that the company was abandoning its stem cell research program due to future financial considerations (Pollack 2011). This unexpected development has been touted in the media as a setback for embryonic stem cell research. Regardless of whether this setback is real or merely perceived, the sudden and premature end to the Geron trial raises ethical concerns regarding the five spinal cord–injury patients who received Geron's stem cell–based transplants, and I shall return to these issues later.

Geron and ACT were the first companies to conduct human studies using embryonic stem cell–derived biologics, but they will surely not be the last. Presently there are several more stem cell–based clinical trials developing along the clinical translation pipeline, so it is fair to say that the era of testing new stem cell–based interventions in human subjects is only just beginning.[7] Among the hES cell–derived therapies now under preclinical development are interventions for diabetes, stroke, and a host of eye disorders. Cellular derivatives of iPS cells are also now being developed to address epidermolysis bullosa, which is a group of inherited disorders that cause severe blistering of the skin. Multipotent stem cell research is also expanding and is just beginning to enter clinical trials using donor cells for heart repair, HIV/AIDS, sickle cell disease, solid tumor cancers, multiple sclerosis, and spinal cord injury, to name a few.

As these and other early stage studies become widely known to the public, there will undoubtedly be much public scrutiny and patient interest in stem cell–based clinical trials. Thus the perspectives of patients and of society will continue to be of importance for the future support of the stem cell field, and I shall return to these perspectives again later. Next, however, I wish to shift our attention to those who are responsible for administering stem cell–based clinical trials. Who are the individuals administering these scientific trials?

The answer is not as simple as it might be in the case of time trials or even criminal trials, where the trial administrators are clearly separate from those who have a personal vested interest in the outcome. Among the individuals administering stem cell–based clinical trials are clinician-scientists and other stem cell researchers; federal, state, or private funders; and regulators from human subject protection committees, federal food and drug agencies, and data and safety monitoring boards.

---

[7] Many of these disease-related research programs are being sponsored by the California Institute for Regenerative Medicine and may be found on their website http://www.cirm.ca.gov/. Furthermore, a recent search of the U.S. government-sponsored website www.clinicaltrials.gov reveals almost 4,000 trials currently involving multipotent cells, mostly hematopoietic and mesenchymal stem cells (accessed April 12, 2012).

In short, the administration of a stem cell–based clinical trial is a collective effort involving many individuals, some of whom may have a personal interest in the outcome of the trial. As a result, the "administrative point of view" is not a singular perspective but rather a knotted assemblage of many vantage points. Each of the various parties involved is faced with many complex challenges and uncertainties, and it will take a bit of effort in the next section to unpack these difficulties and bring them to light. It is imperative, however, that patients and society at large be made aware of these technical and ethical issues.

## The Challenges Facing Stem Cell–Based Clinical Trials

Everything I have suggested thus far about the views of patients, society, and trial administrators could be applied to most clinical trials conducted in other areas of biomedicine. Nevertheless, our need to consider each of these perspectives is heightened by the novel nature of stem cell–based therapies and their potentially transformative impact on modern medicine. Expanding on this assertion, I want first to bring to the reader's attention some important features of stem cell–based medical interventions that might make it difficult for them to fit seamlessly into the current clinical trials system.

Traditionally, the clinical trials process originated for the regulatory purposes of developing pharmaceutical drugs for marketing and human use. There are four phases in the clinical trials process.[8] Phase I clinical trials assess the safety of an investigational product in a small number of human subjects. Normally, human subjects enrolled in Phase I studies are healthy volunteers or patients for whom there are no other effective treatments available. If there are no major adverse events at Phase I then investigators can proceed to the next step. Phase II trials aim at assessing the efficacy of the medical product in larger numbers of human subjects, usually ranging from ten to more than a hundred patients who have medical conditions relevant to the product. Many investigational products fail at this stage because they do not demonstrate their anticipated effects, are not well tolerated by patients, or do not perform favorably compared to current treatments. The few medical products that pass this phase of testing then proceed to the next phase. Phase III clinical trials involve testing the investigational product on large groups of patient

---

[8] A good summary of this phased process can be found at www.clinicaltrials.gov (accessed April 12, 2012).

research subjects (up to several thousand) to corroborate its effectiveness and to monitor further its safety and side effects. Most investigational products flounder at this stage of research due to the enormous financial expense of conducting Phase III trials and because investigators often fail to enroll enough human subjects for their study. In the United States, Phase III clinical trials are especially significant because this is the final testing stage before product registration. Investigational products that pass Phase III trials are approved by federal regulators for marketed patient use. Finally, in some cases, an approved medical product will proceed to Phase IV, which are postapproval trials conducted after entry into the marketplace for ongoing safety monitoring and for understanding the product's optimal use.

Passage through the clinical trials process is an arduous undertaking, and the vast majority of investigational drugs fail to make it all the way through from first-in-human studies to final regulatory approval. From 1991 to 2000, only 11 percent of all new pharmaceutical drugs were approved by European and/or U.S. regulatory agencies (Kola and Landis 2004). In light of this high attrition rate, two drug industry leaders have offered a series of practical recommendations to guide investigators toward successful product development: (1) investigators must show very strong evidence of proof of mechanism; (2) must rule out any compounds that have mechanism-based toxicity by using preclinical toxicity studies; (3) should identify biomarkers that signify correct dosing; (4) need to pay very close attention to the design of first-in-human clinical studies so that they might capture some evidence of efficacy rather than waiting to establish efficacy later in far more expensive trial phases; (5) must design their human studies based on appropriate efficacy testing in animal models; and (6) investigators and sponsors should be wary of the possibility that their investigational product may not be commercially competitive, either because it compares unfavorably to other drugs further along in development or because their product is not much different from what is available (Kola and Landis 2004). Each of these recommendations makes excellent sense; however, none is effortless or uncomplicated. This is especially true for the development of stem cell–based biologics.

I explained in Chapter 2 that stem cell–based biologics are not like pharmaceutical drugs. Unlike pills, which are stable and easily defined by their chemical properties, stem cells and their derivatives are living, dynamic entities with an astounding degree of plasticity. I had argued that the plasticity of stem cells in culture is a capacity that is neither fully natural nor fully artificial; rather, stem cell plasticity is produced by the combination of cell-intrinsic biological properties plus laboratory intervention and human artifice. In most cases, stem cells and their direct derivatives are completely novel products for which manufacturing processes and standards for safety, purity, potency, and genetic stability are not yet fully established (International Society for Stem Cell Research 2008a). Take the case of iPS cells. It bears mentioning that direct reprogramming affects the somatic cell nuclear genome but not the mitochondria, and it is unclear at this point whether aged or altered mitochondria will affect the biological characteristics of iPS cells and their direct derivatives (Koch et al. 2009). I believe uncertainties such as this come from the fact that stem cells and their derivatives reside somewhere along a broad continuum spanning the wholly natural and the wholly artificial, depending on the cell type in question and the laboratory techniques used to generate and/or sustain it. Attempting to address important questions for product development, such as mechanism of action, mechanism-based toxicity, and correct dosing, can be a far more elusive task than if stem cell–based products were either completely natural entities, like organs and donor tissues, or completely man-made, like pills.

Furthermore, animal models do not often fully mirror the complex human diseases targeted by stem cell–based interventions, making efficacy, toxicity, immune responses, and other biologic responses in humans difficult to predict. Some stem cell–based interventions must be tested in large animal models, and there are no simple or appropriate means for imaging stem cell–derived transplants in large live animals to track where the cells go and how well they survive and function. And even if functionally accurate imaging instruments could be devised for large animal models, the very notion of cell potency (i.e., the degree to which a manufactured cell produces its desired effect) is a purely retrospective determination. That is part of the trouble with cell potency. The cells researchers use to determine potency in animal models are not, strictly speaking, the same cells that will go into the patient. Thus there will always be uncertainty, because the only experiment that will provide clarity regarding true potency is the one conducted in the patient, although as before, potency will be retrospectively shown if the experiment works at all.[9] So although preclinical safety and efficacy testing in animals is highly desirable, stem cell investigators may often have to proceed to first-in-human clinical trials without complete knowledge of human toxicity, mechanism of action, or effectiveness.

---

[9]  I thank Willy Lensch for raising this issue about human cell potency assays using animal models.

I have suggested that it may be quite difficult for stem cell investigators to fulfill recommendations one through five previously outlined. What about recommendation six? Stem cell researchers and product developers should abide by the suggestion that they keep their eye on making their stem cell–based intervention commercially and clinically competitive. Stem cell–based therapies should aim to be more efficacious than other treatment alternatives and/or provide cost-effective advantages, such as one-time administration versus lifelong drug therapy with associated side effects and steep long-term costs. Many people believe that one of the major potential advantages of stem cell–based transplant therapies is that they could persist in patients for many years and provide very long-term health benefits. However, to establish that the benefits of a stem cell therapy are long lasting, investigators and sponsors face the practical difficulty of having to wait many years to show that this is actually the case. In the meantime, competing, more conventional chemical approaches to treating disease may speed ahead toward regulatory approval.

One can see from these discussions that the road to stem cell clinical translation is long, complex, and unpredictable. In addition to the issues mentioned, it is also important to reiterate that the administration of the clinical trials process is a very interactive one, and that the administrative perspective is not comprised of just one party's point of view. As stem cell investigators advance new stem cell–based therapies toward clinical trials, they will have to negotiate additional issues with their sponsors and regulators. For example, federal regulators in the United States require that the biologic product used in human trials must be identical to the product that was used in all the preclinical work necessary to justify entry into a Phase I trial. Thus, in the case of Geron, for example, the company had to scale up the production of their hES cell–derived oligodendroglial progenitor cells (a biologic product it named GRNOPC1) to support more than forty separate animal studies.[10] Eventually, after frequent consultations with federal regulatory officials, Geron ended up submitting an investigational new drug application to the U.S. FDA which was over twenty-two thousand pages long.

At this point one may begin to wonder exactly *what* is undergoing the clinical trials process. From the point of view of regulators, investigators, and sponsors, the answer may be that it is the *biologic product* that is undergoing testing. After all, the product is the subject of the

---

[10] Personal communication with Catherine Priest, Geron.

investigational new drug application, and it is the product that the sponsors and researchers have to worry about in terms of scaling up and maintaining quality, consistency, and the like. In listening to scientific presentations about new stem cell–based products under development, I have always been struck by the way in which animal and human research subjects are often portrayed as *in vivo* testing platforms for the product. Most of these discussions have focused on the preclinical scientific and regulatory requirements that are necessary to bring a stem cell–based intervention to the point of study in humans. Human trials represent the final steps in the product's journey to the clinic. Thus, from the point of view of funders, investigators, and regulators, who together must administer stem cell–based clinical trials, it is easy to see why one might answer that it is the *product* that is undergoing these trials.[11]

But human research subjects are not simply performance-testing platforms for new stem cell technologies. This is true for two reasons. The first reason is obvious. Human research subjects are persons who morally deserve to be treated in a way that respects their capacity for autonomy and for whom clinicians have a professional ethical duty not to harm. We already saw in Chapters 3 and 4 how research ethics deal with this first point through the philosophical values of respect for persons, beneficence, and justice, and through the corresponding practical doctrines of informed consent, reasonable risk-benefit ratios for research participation, and fair subject selection. I do not mean to suggest here that most scientists have a disrespectful or dismissive attitude toward human participants in research – that they see human subjects as mere tools for product development and regulatory approval. I have met many clinician-scientists who emphatically do not harbor these views. However, many scientists do seem to believe that concerns about how to ethically manage human research subjects should be left mainly up to research oversight committees.

This last response, however typical it may be, still does not address the second reason why one should not view human research subjects as mere testing platforms for new biologics. Stem cell–based interventions involve a series of very close biological interactions between the cell product

---

[11] It is worth noting that from a public point of view it may actually be the stem cell biotech company (such as Geron or ACT) that is being tested in a clinical trial, or, perhaps much more broadly, the field of embryonic stem cell research. The success or failure of a trial may signify to many observers success or failure of a company or an area of research. This latter point was well illustrated in the case of gene transfer research with the death of Jesse Gelsinger in 1999.

and the patient's local and/or systemic biological attributes. The necessary mutual responses between the intervention and the patient's body make it difficult to justify the simple view that it is merely the product that is undergoing testing in humans. According to my analysis, it is the product and the human subject *together as one unit* that is being tested. I believe patients, investigators, regulators, and others must remain mindful of this point. The biological interdependence between product and patient has ethical implications for clinical trial design, which I explain over the course of the next two sections.

## Guidelines for Stem Cell–Based Clinical Trials

It is widely acknowledged that clinical trials may pose many unknown risks for human subjects, especially first-in-human studies (Solbakk and Zoloth 2011). In light of the preceding discussions, it is fair to say that stem cell–based clinical trials can carry risks that are especially grave and unknown. Among these risks are the risk of tumor formation (if the biologic product is contaminated with undifferentiated stem cells); unwanted cell proliferation, migration, and overgrowth; and immune rejection of donated cell populations.[12] There may also be the risk of opportunity costs for patients who are enrolled in the experimental arm of a stem cell–based clinical trial and so do not receive all standard therapies.

In light of these risks and many other challenges facing the clinical translation of stem cells, the ISSCR convened an international task force of experts to produce professional guidelines to help transition basic stem cell research into appropriate applications for patients (Hyun et al. 2008; International Society for Stem Cell Research 2008a).[13] Large portions of the ISSCR's clinical translation guidelines have been devoted to topics that I have already discussed, such as cell processing and manufacture and preclinical research. Other portions of the guidelines address medical innovation and stem cell tourism, which I discuss in Chapter 8. In this section I wish to direct the reader's attention to what

---

[12] E.g., a preclinical study conducted in Germany revealed that when mesenchymal stem cells (MSCs) were injected into mouse models of myocardial infarction, the MSCs turned into bone 51.2% of the time (Breitbach et al. 2007).

[13] This international task force was comprised of scientists, surgeons, gene transfer researchers, bioethicists, patient advocates, and attorneys. Readers can access multiple translations of the ISSCR's *Guidelines for the Clinical Translation of Stem Cells* at www.isscr.org (accessed August 4, 2011).

the guidelines recommend for the ethical treatment of human subjects in stem cell–based clinical trials. These recommendations represent the first of their kind for the stem cell field, and for that reason alone they are quite significant.

The ISSCR clinical translation guidelines state that clinical trials involving the direct derivatives of pluripotent stem cells or novel uses of multipotent stem cells must be reviewed and approved by local human protections committees. These ethics committees (IRBs or other equivalent ethics review boards) should include individuals with the supplemental scientific expertise necessary to evaluate the unique biological aspects of stem cell–based products. The ISSCR guidelines call for the rigorous review of any proposals aiming to test novel stem cell–based treatments in patients, with expert judgments made about the reliability and rigor of any preclinical evidence to support one's proceeding to a human study. All committee reviews must be conducted independently of the investigators' influence, and all reviews must ensure that research subjects are making voluntary and informed decisions to participate.

In order to promote voluntary informed consent, the ISSCR guidelines recommend that the unique risks of stem cell–based interventions be communicated clearly to all potential research subjects. For example, patients must be informed of whether the stem cell–based product has ever been tested before in humans and whether there are any unknown physical risks.[14] Potential research subjects need to understand that stem cell–based products are not like pharmaceutical drugs or implanted medical devices which can be withdrawn from subjects if adverse reactions occur. Stem cell–based products may not leave the subjects body and may cause ill effects on the patient for the rest of his or her life.[15]

---

[14] Investigators must be very careful how they describe their stem cell–based product during subject recruitment for clinical trials. According to the accepted terminology for engineered tissues developed by the Division for Tissue Engineered Medical Products of the American Society for Testing and Materials, the term *equivalent* cell types should not be used in reference to any engineered tissue. Rather, one should use the term *tissue substitute* instead (www.astm.org; accessed April 19, 2012) I raise this point to highlight my concern that, by describing a stem cell–based product as being "equivalent" to another cell type (such as oligodendroglial progenitor cells), investigators may inadvertently mislead potential research subjects into thinking that these manufactured cells are the same as cells found during the course of normal human development. No one knows for sure whether manufactured cells from stem cells are equivalent to natural cell types; therefore, they should not be presented as such.

[15] One often-proposed strategy is to modify stem cell biologics with "suicide genes." These are transferred genes that would make the transplanted cells sensitive to a drug that researchers could administer to selectively kill the stem cell product in the patient's body. However, representatives from the FDA have noted that a suicide gene strategy

Clinician-scientists must evaluate each patient's understanding of these unique risks at the time of their obtaining informed consent for research. This cotemporaneous evaluation should involve a "teach back" method for assessing understanding, either through a short written test or an oral quiz, to determine whether the patient truly comprehends the most crucial talking points covered in the consent process.

The ISSCR guidelines also recommend going beyond the informed consent procedure to manage the ethics of patient research participation. The guidelines place the responsibility for the welfare of human subjects also on clinical trial administrators. For example, researchers, funders, and regulators alike must insist on long-term health monitoring of research subjects and must make available to subjects adequate health insurance coverage or medical resources to cover any research-related complications. Trial administrators must also have a clear action plan for adverse event reporting and treatment for research-related injuries. And all clinical trials must be monitored by independent data and safety monitoring boards.

In short, the ISSCR guidelines for clinical translation address the ethics of human subjects research in ways that are typical for other fields of biomedical research, but with added emphasis on the unique risks of stem cell–based therapies. Chief among these risks are the unknown ill effects of long-lasting stem cell–based transplants and possibility of very long-term patient involvement. These special issues require us to think very carefully about the ethics of clinical trial design and risk-benefit ratios for first-in-human trials. The ISSCR guidelines give us a very good starting point for doing this; however, they should be supplemented with further consideration of these latter two points.

## Issues in Trial Design

Some stem cell–based therapies could, in principle, produce lifelong benefits for patients. We know this to be the case when we consider the most widely used stem cell–based clinical therapy today – hematopoietic stem cell transplantation for blood disorders – an intervention that offers a lifetime cure for many patients receiving donor grafts.[16] Furthermore,

---

might raise risks for human subjects in other ways so that the overall balance of risk may not be improved. The best approach would be to ensure that there are no unwanted cells in the biologic product. FDA official, personal communication.

[16] Hematopoietic stem cells, which are the therapeutic components of whole bone marrow and umbilical cord blood, have been shown to be effective for treating genetic blood disorders like thalassemia and immune deficiency and cancers like leukemia and

it has been reported that some Parkinson's disease patients in Sweden who received neural transplants of human fetal dopaminergic neurons showed signs of clinical benefit more fifteen years posttransplant (Lindvall et al. 2004; Piccini et al. 1999).[17] The possibility of long-lasting or even lifetime engraftment makes the design of stem cell–based clinical trials especially challenging. In this section I use the example of cell therapy for Parkinson's disease to illustrate many of these trial design challenges.[18]

Experiences with cell therapy for Parkinson's disease suggest that the stage of disease and the study endpoints of a clinical trial are crucial. Inspired in part by the reports coming out of Sweden, two American NIH-funded sham surgery-controlled trials were conducted to evaluate the effectiveness of fetal-derived dopaminergic neuron grafting for Parkinson's disease (Freed et al. 2001; Olanow et al. 2003). The authors of the first study concluded that, after one year, human embryonic dopamine-neuron transplants survived in patients with severe Parkinson's disease and produced some clinical benefit for younger patients, but not for patients over the age of sixty (Freed et al. 2001). The authors of the second study concluded that there were no significant overall treatment effects of transplanting fetal dopaminergic neurons in Parkinson's

lymphoma. It should be acknowledged, however, that roughly 50% of patients receiving hematopoietic stem cells are not cured or are left with permanent disabilities. George Daley, personal communication.

It is also interesting to note that the first reported cases of bone marrow transplant by Edward Donnall Thomas in the late 1950s involved not clinical trials but rather clinically innovative interventions for gravely ill patients with few medical alternatives (Thomas 1999; Thomas et al. 1957). All of these patients died soon after treatment. In 1990, Thomas shared the Nobel Prize in Medicine with Joseph Murray, the surgeon who performed the first successful human kidney transplant in 1954. It is worth acknowledging that these early advances in hematopoietic stem cell and kidney transplantation did not occur within the context of clinical trials. I explore in Chapter 8 the ethics of stem cell–based medical innovations outside clinical trials.

[17] One of the major disadvantages of transplanting fetal dopaminergic neurons is the heterogeneity of the donor samples, possibly leading to uneven clinical outcomes across patients. Thus researchers are seeking ways to derive much more uniform, transplantable dopaminergic neurons derived from human pluripotent stem cells. Olle Lindvall, personal communication.

[18] My analysis here is aimed primarily at clinical trials for stem cell–based transplantation therapies and not other types of therapies that might use stem cells or their derivatives like drugs to transiently stimulate endogenous healing support around an injury. See Chapter 2 for a discussion of the various types of stem cell–based intervention strategies. Stem cell–based transplantation therapies are especially promising for medical conditions where the defects are largely constrained to the cellular level such that restoration of function through cell replacement could cure patients or greatly relieve their symptoms.

disease patients and that, based on their results, they could not recommend this intervention as a therapy for Parkinson's (Olanow et al. 2003). Swedish researchers responded to these studies by pointing out that only short-term or no immunosuppression was given to these patients, and that immune reactions may have caused graft dysfunction (Lindvall et al. 2004). Furthermore, the patients in the American studies were more severely disabled at the time of transplantation than the patients in the Swedish studies, thus suggesting that dopaminergic neuron transplantation was not as effective for extensive degeneration. It is interesting to note, however, that the authors of the first study followed their patients subjects for four years posttransplantation and were surprised to discover that many patients had even more significant improvements after the one-year time point of their original published article. The researchers reported that, in posttransplant year two, the younger Parkinson's disease patients had twice the improvement over year one. And by year four many of the older patients caught up to many of the younger patients (Ma et al. 2010). These results seem to agree with the results of the Swedish studies that dopeminergic neuron grafting for Parkinson's disease can produce long-lasting clinical benefits that increase over time, although graft-induced dyskinesias (involuntary motions) continued to be a problem for some patients.

The previously mentioned Parkinson's disease example instructs us to pay attention to the following issues. The first is the problem of what type of subjects ought to be recruited for first-in-human stem cell studies. Normally in Phase I toxicity studies of pharmaceutical drugs, investigators use a small number of healthy volunteers or severely ill patients with few alternatives. For stem cell–based therapies, however, it makes little sense to administer a stem cell–based biologic to healthy volunteers, because these biologic products will not interact in the right way with healthy individuals, and in many cases the biologic may not be able to be safely removed. So investigators must use research subjects recruited from a relevant patient population, especially one for whom the possibly of a long-lasting, integrative transplant may be more acceptable. But at what stage of the disease process ought one to attempt the investigational intervention?

Ethically, one might propose that the best patient subjects are those who are near the end of their disease course for whom all other conventional therapies have failed. Such patients may have the "least to lose" in participating in a Phase I trial. But from a scientific point of view this population may not be ideal, because early phase stem cell–based clinical trials may show negligible or zero therapeutic effect in very seriously ill patients. Additionally, if the aim of the investigational intervention is to slow down a degenerative disease process, then testing the intervention in seriously ill patients would be counterintuitive. By contrast, using patients for a Phase I clinical trial who are in early disease stages also poses problems, because such patients typically have good therapeutic alternatives at that time which can ameliorate their symptoms and provide a reasonable quality of life for many years, as is the case with L-dopa therapy and deep brain stimulation (DBS) for Parkinson's disease. The ethical challenge then in many Phase I stem cell–based clinical trials is how to justify recruiting relatively well-off patients diagnosed with a degenerative disease when their enrollment may expose them to known risks (such as graft-induced dyskinesias) and other unknown short-term and long-term risks, including possible limitations on their ability to receive proven, conventional therapies.

In addition to deciding which type of patients to enroll, investigators and regulators must also decide the correct temporal and efficacy endpoints for the study. These endpoints are crucial, for they help set the parameters for evaluating the success of a trial. Should the efficacy endpoint be to demonstrate safety only, or should the Phase I trial also demonstrate survival and appropriate cell behavior of the transplanted product in patients?[19] Should physiotherapy be included as part of the cell therapy? Should global measures be included, such as whether the patient subject reports feeling better? What about clinical measures, such as, in the case of Parkinson's disease, the Unified Parkinson's Disease Rating Scale? And how long should the study last? Most Phase I clinical trials last one year. But as we saw in the preceding text in the case of Parkinson's disease, cell-based therapies showed greater improvement for patients in year two and beyond. Stopping the study at year one to compare results with the control group and/or with standard therapies may not provide a good picture of what a cell-based therapy is truly capable of achieving. It could be the case that, in Parkinson's disease and other degenerative diseases, a stem cell–based therapy could produce benefits at an increasing rate over a longer period or have a small effect in the short term but a much large effect in the long term after further cell engraftment and proliferation. Moreover, how one defines *efficacy* matters in terms of what measurement standards one intends to employ.

---

[19] The primary endpoint in the Geron spinal cord–injury trial was safety after one year posttransplant. The secondary endpoint was some evidence of change in function.

Therefore, efficacy and temporal endpoints are extremely important for determining the success of a stem cell–based therapy. Unfortunately there are no obvious answers for what these endpoints ought to be.

Not only are the endpoints important but so are the comparators. What should be the controls in a stem cell–based clinical trial? The answer will depend in large part on the specifics of the phase of the clinical trials process, the nature of the stem cell–based intervention, the nature of the disease, and the treatment alternatives and standard of care available for patients. These are very complex considerations to take into account, so the answer will never be easy or uncontroversial. For example, it has been widely debated whether sham surgery is justified in cell-based clinical trials for Parkinson's disease, with up to 94 percent of North American researchers favoring the practice and many bioethicists railing against it for imposing unnecessary risks on research subjects (Kim et al. 2005; Macklin 1999). The two American studies referenced in the preceding text used sham surgery with double blinding (a procedure that involves administering burr holes in the skulls of patients in the placebo group and leaving it unknown to patients and researchers regarding which individuals received cell transplants and which received nothing).

In contrast, most Parkinson's disease researchers in Europe tend to be strongly against sham surgery. Clinical neuroscientist Roger Barker has argued that sham controls provide very little statistical utility in studies in which the numbers of research subjects are quite small, as is the case with the early phases of cell-based therapy trials (Katsnelson 2011). Barker has suggested instead that an observational study could be used wherein a group of early onset Parkinson's disease patients could be asked whether they want the cell-based experimental intervention or standard therapy. Researchers would let the patients choose for themselves and then track all of them.[20] Instead of using sham controls with double blinding, in which case neither the subjects nor the researchers know who is in the control group, Barker's proposed approach would be to use an open-label study where patients and clinician-scientists are aware that every subject has received cell transplants. This approach may have the added ethical advantage that – unlike subjects in a blinded, sham controlled trial – patients would not have to expend a great deal of mental energy stressing over whether they received a cell transplant, only to be disappointed or discouraged later when they are unblinded and discover they were assigned to the placebo group.

---

[20] Roger Barker, personal communication.

Besides the issue of whether to use sham control groups, there are important questions about the right sample size of patient research subjects at all phases of the clinical trials system. The first concern is this. Stem cell and other cell-based interventions such as fetal dopaminergic neuron grafting are invasive, so only a few patients ought to be enrolled during the early phases of research. But given this small sample size, there is a very limited capacity to assess efficacy, and one cannot really assess safety. To rule out whether an intervention produces an unintended bad effect, researchers must study a very large sample size. Sometimes the adverse side effects of a new drug are not fully known until after that drug has been approved for patient use and is distributively marketed to a very large number of people. Given these statistical constraints and realities, it is extremely difficult to interpret the results of early studies using small numbers of patients. Unfortunately, there are also sample-size problems for later phases in the clinical trials process designed to help address these earlier statistical challenges. It may be unrealistic for regulators to expect that a stem cell–based therapy (especially one involving a very complex manufactured biologic product) can feasibly be tested in thousands of patients in late Phase II and early Phase III trials. This is a point that might require negotiation because financial sponsors may be unable to support the production of so many investigational product samples. How can this negotiation of sample size proceed while preserving the need for good scientific evidence?

None of these questions has an easy solution, for each is intertwined with the others in a manner that defies an easy systematic approach. For example, if the efficacy endpoint of a trial is to delay the onset of a later stage in a degenerative disease process – such as the H&Y stage 3 onset of balance impairment in Parkinson's disease (Hoehn and Yahr 1967) – then the ages of the patient research subjects matter. Researchers may not want to try a cell-based intervention on young Parkinson's disease patients who are early in the disease process, because there may be no difference in outcome when compared to Parkinson's disease patients getting the best available care. If a cell-based therapy such as dopaminergic neuron grafting is compared to a standard therapy, such as DBS, the former is likely to lose in the comparison when the subject groups involve young patients. Thus the selection of subjects, stage of disease, and definition of *efficacy* all intersect as problems.[21]

---

[21] Ibid.

Finally, we must consider the difficult issue of responsible subject withdrawal from a study. What does it mean to withdraw a patient subject from a stem cell–based clinical trial, especially when the biologic product has been deeply integrated within the patient's body? What if the patient wishes to drop out of the study and wants to have the integrated biologic product removed? Assuming that product can be purged from the body, what would be the correct course of action if, in the opposite scenario, researchers or regulators halt the trial for safety reasons but the patient refuses to have the stem cell–based biologic removed? Exactly who owns the biologically integrated product? These are important issues to address in advance, because subject withdrawal might entail not only cell removal but also an end to patient monitoring and responsibility. As the Geron spinal cord–injury trial illustrates, it is not just researchers and regulators that can halt a study but funders as well. It is unclear at the time of this writing exactly who is responsible for the five paralyzed patients whose spines have been injected with Geron's biologic product GRNOPC1. Whether a study has been halted or has run its proposed course, there should be a clear plan for long-term health monitoring and follow-up. This raises the question of who should be the physician in charge after the study is over. Who should be responsible for the patient's ongoing care?

As the preceding discussions show, the task of designing a clinical trial for stem cell–based clinical therapies is challenged by uncertain standards and conflicting values. Decisions have to be made about at which stage of the disease process to test the intervention, what to define as the temporal and efficacy endpoints, what controls to use, and so forth. These open-ended issues carry different trade-offs depending on what standards of evaluation are selected. This open-endedness – the modulation of which researchers, funders, regulators, and other administrators must constantly negotiate – should be surprising to those who assume that any type of trial must have clearly defined boundaries, such as unambiguous endpoints and widely agreed-upon standards of evaluation. In this way, clinical trials are definitely not like time trials. The administration of a stem cell–based clinical trial is an interactive, multiperspectival process of negotiation. If this is admittedly the case, then why not also include the perspectives of patients and patient groups in trial design?

We can tick off some quick reasons why including patient perspectives would be a good idea. First, patients' priorities and their standards of evaluation and success may be quite different from those of researchers and administrators. For example, according to a poll of Parkinson's disease patients spanning thirty-one European countries, being able to sleep through the night, feeling less tired, and not having to plan one's life around a strict medication schedule all ranked very high on a list of patient priorities (http://www.epda.eu.com; accessed April 10, 2012). Based on these types of preferences, patients might select different efficacy endpoints than those defined by researchers and others not experienced in living with the disease. Deep brain stimulation is frequently identified by clinicians and regulators as an effective therapy for ameliorating many Parkinson's disease patients' symptoms. However, it is possible that some patients may prefer to have more choices available to them, including cell-based therapies, even if DBS is shown to be more effective in the short term for maintaining motor control.[22]

Second, by including patient perspectives one may be able to improve the informed consent process for research. Rather than simply imagining what patients may need to know for the consent interview, it may be far more effective for researchers and regulators to ask patients directly what they actually need to know to make a clear and informed decision. Empirical sociological research has already shown that asking patient decision makers how to improve informed consent for Phase I leukemia trials has led to dramatically different and much more informative consent procedures (Eder et al. 2007). I believe the same is likely to hold true for stem cell–based clinical trials.

The preceding considerations provide good, practice-driven rationales for including patient perspectives. I believe, however, that there is an additional, much more philosophical reason for promoting such patient inclusiveness. By doing so we might help address the incommensurability problem surrounding the design of stem cell–based clinical trials.

## The Incommensurability Problem Revisited

I had introduced the incommensurability problem in Chapter 3, where I suggested it might pose a difficulty for philosophical research ethics. I proposed that the incommensurability of the four core moral values supporting ethical research (i.e., scientific integrity, beneficence, respect for persons, and justice) may preclude the possibility of there being a justifiable way to balance each of these values against the others. In this section I discuss the challenge that incommensurability presents to the ethical design and administration of stem cell–based clinical trials.

---

[22] Ibid.

Incommensurability results when the values of different aims or goods cannot be reduced to a common measure for comparison and choice. In cases of true incommensurability (as opposed to the practical incompatibility of not being able to have one's cake and eat it too), the value of each option cannot be placed on the same scale of measurement without grossly distorting our understanding of what it means for each option to be valuable in its distinct way. For example, one may propose that mercy and justice are incommensurable, and so are knowledge and happiness, liberty and filial duty, and so forth. Each of these aims is valuable and worth pursuing in its own right. But their corresponding goodness or worth cannot be compared along a single scale so that we know rationally what the magnitudes of the trade-offs are when they clash. Take the following examples. In times of conflict, which is greater – extending the duration of a patient's life in an ICU or maintaining the quality of that patient's life at the end of her disease course? In health-care policy setting, which is greater – giving priority to historically disadvantaged populations in greatest need of health-care resources or to populations that (because they are already socially advantaged) stand to gain the greatest health benefits per dollar? In autonomous decision making, which is greater – a young man's civic duty to join the Free French Forces or his filial duty to stay home to care for his ailing mother (Sartre 1946)? Whether we are talking about end-of-life decision making, health resource priority setting, or the personal conflicts of Jean-Paul Sartre's idealistic young man in 1940s France, the incommensurability of life's options entails that our tragic choice of one worthy option over another leaves us with a sense of uncompensated loss. This sense of loss seems to sharpen, not ease, when we concede that there appears to be no rational way for us to choose between incommensurables.

We face the same type of incommensurability problem when we ponder the conflicting values at stake in stem cell–based clinical trials. In most clinical trial situations – particularly first-in-human studies and other very early clinical trials phases – researchers, regulators, and other trial administrators are required to weigh (a) the potential physical, psychological, social, and economic harms to the research subject against (b) the potential gains in scientific knowledge and broad social benefit. Because early stage clinical trials aim primarily at assessing safety rather than efficacy, researchers usually do not have to justify their trial by comparing *ex ante* the plurality of possible harms for each research subject against a slim possibility of subject benefit (although this scenario presents its own incommensurability problem – the issue of comparing for each individual a range of qualitatively different harms and benefits as if one were able to compare apples to oranges to bananas to pears). Instead, decision makers must weigh the subject's possible research-related harms against a host of potential downstream benefits to science and society – benefits that can be aggregated across many individuals. This presents the difficulty of trying to compare apples and so forth to haystacks. If the bearers of value on either side of the risk-benefit ratio are not reducible to a common unit of measurement – that is, not reducible without significantly distorting our understanding of these bearers of value (such as patient subject well-being vs. scientific and social benefit) – then we do not seem to have a justified means for comparing and balancing the two sides of the scale.

Some philosophers might argue that any bearers of value can be analyzable for our balancing purposes if we reduce their worth down to uniform increments of "utility" as defined by various strains of utilitarian ethics. However, assuming that this could be done without gross distortion (and I am very doubtful of this), we come face-to-face with the aggregation effect. The aggregation effect is the conclusion that any small number of individuals will have their interests overwhelmed each time their interests are measured in terms of utilities found in far greater quantities in a much larger group. If utilitarians succeed in translating all competing values into heaps of uniform units of utility, then larger heaps will always outweigh smaller heaps – social benefit and scientific advancement will always triumph over the possible harms (loss of benefits) to a few research subjects. So we are either faced with an unresolved incommensurability problem, or we can resolve the conflict between individual harms and social and scientific advancement by simply forcing everything onto a common scale of utilities and assigning the losing side of the equation to individual research subjects every time.

Other philosophers may point out, however, that it is not really incommensurability we should worry about but rather incomparability. Incommensurability occurs when there is no common unit of measurement against which we can rationally base our comparisons and decisions. But this lack need not preclude our ability to make comparisons among options (Chang 1997). Commensurability, some would argue, matters only if we are interested in cardinal rankings, that is, rankings based on some uniform numerical scale, such as the heights in meters of various mountaintops in the French Pyrenees. Perhaps all we really need is just a way to make ordinal rankings – that is, rough and less precise rankings in an order of first, second, and third place, such as the final placement list of contestants in a beauty pageant. Some philosophers maintain that all we need to know is roughly which options are good, better, and best relative to one another; we do not need cardinal precision about what numerical values can be calculated to produce a final rank order. If it is true that ordinal ranking is what ultimately matters for our discussion, then we may still be able to make justified comparisons between different alternatives that are incommensurable. How is this possible?

One leading philosophical explanation is that comparisons between two incommensurable goods can be achieved if these comparisons are made in terms of some "covering value" that holds between them (Chang 1997). Such comparisons will take the form "*X* is better than *Y* with respect to covering value *V*." For example, one might argue that a legal career is better than an artistic career with respect to income, even though the value of law and art are incommensurable, or that doing philosophy is better than bowling with respect to the engagement of one's higher-order mental faculties, even though, as John Stuart Mill would declare, there is no single quality of pleasure that is common across both philosophy and bowling. If this approach is correct, then it is incomparability not incommensurability that we should be worried about in our discussion of stem cell–based clinical trials. To say that two alternatives are *incomparable* is a different and much stronger claim than saying that they are *incommensurable*, for incomparability means that there is no covering value whatsoever that holds between them, that is, no positive value relation with respect to which a meaningful evaluative comparison can ever be made. On this analysis, the incommensurability problem may simply fade into irrelevance, not to be replaced by any other chief difficulty. On this analysis, the possibility of a justified choice between competing alternatives is not precluded, so long as these alternatives are comparable in terms of at least one covering value.

Unfortunately, I do not believe shifting our focus from incommensurability to incomparability helps us analyze the trade-offs involved in stem cell–based clinical trials. For one, this philosophical strategy transforms the incommensurability problem into a different but still difficult problem of identifying and, more importantly, justifying which covering value or values we ought to employ to balance (for example) the value of scientific integrity and social beneficence against the different potential harms facing patient research subjects. What covering values are up to this task? I cannot come up with one that is adequate. For instance, what is the covering value for comparing (a) the badness of graft-induced dyskinesias for patients participating in a Parkinson's disease clinical trial to

(b) the goodness of learning more about the scientific promise of dopaminergic cell-based therapies? Does (b) take precedence over (a) or is (a) more significant than (b)? On the basis of what covering value can we make such a determination? Can we find appropriate covering values to settle other examples of incommensurability we considered earlier? What is the covering value for justice and mercy, knowledge and happiness, liberty and filial duty? I am skeptical there is a satisfactory answer for any of these cases, much less a straightforward way to rationalize our choice of which covering value is appropriate to ground the comparison. I am suspicious that, in many practical situations, our covering value – that is, our overarching standard providing the comparative basis for evaluation – may simply amount to a bias or prejudice masquerading as a justifying reason to rank one alternative ordinally above another. If covering values justify our choice between incommensurables, then what justifies our choice of covering values, yet another covering value? I leave it up to the reader to contemplate these philosophical indeterminacies further.[23]

There is one more odd feature of the covering value approach that merits mentioning. The strategy of shifting our focus from incommensurability to incomparability seems to overlook the important fact that the potential harms to the research subject and the potential benefits to science and society are scalar – that the types of harms and benefits in question each have magnitudes. Harms come in degrees, and so do benefits. In comparing possible benefits and harms (understood perhaps as benefits lost) it matters to our decision making what the magnitudes of these benefits and harms are. Curiously, the covering value approach appears to be insensitive to the scalar properties of harms and benefits. The formulation "*X* is better than *Y* with respect to covering value *V*"

---

[23] There are other philosophers who maintain that some noncomparative considerations can justify one's choice, even if one's alternatives are incommensurable and incomparable. For instance, prudence, as well as legal or moral consensus, might provide one's choice with some justificatory standards (Griffin 1997). Or a choice for A over B could be justified on the ground that A is good on some absolute, noncomparative evaluative standard (Stocker 1997). Or choices might be justified by one's lived experience (Millgram 1997; Wiggins 1997). I do not have space here to elaborate on these strategies for noncomparative justifications of choice or to explore their weaknesses. Ultimately, I do not believe these approaches resolve the issue we are dealing with in this section – namely, the problem of justifying a choice among incommensurable (perhaps even incomparable) values, particularly in cases in which the decision makers are not the same individuals as those research subjects for whom this balance is being weighed. I touch very briefly on some of this again in the following text when I discuss the limits of institutional or procedural means for dealing with the incommensurability problem.

does nothing to guarantee that the magnitudes of *X* and *Y* are properly taken into account. If the possible individual harms and scientific benefits of an early phase stem cell–based clinical trial are by nature scalar, then incommensurability is the correct concern, not incomparability divorced from the relevance of measurement. Even if we insist on striving for ordinal, not cardinal, rankings, we can always pause to ask the question "if *A* is better than *B*, then how much better is it?" Comparisons of benefits and harms that have scalar properties must involve calculation at some point, and if this is true then we are right back to our original incommensurability problem. Unfortunately, the scalar properties of the various harms and benefits open to research subjects and to society do not seem to be reducible to the same units of value measurement. That, I am afraid, lies at the heart of the incommensurability problem for clinical trials.

Given what I have argued, must we conclude that the incommensurability problem is insurmountable for stem cell–based clinical trials? Is there no basis for justifiably choosing how to balance the potential harms to subjects against the potential benefits for science and society? Perhaps our situation is not so dire. Perhaps a tentative answer to these questions comes from Joseph Raz's approach to incommensurability (Raz 1997). On Raz's view, incommensurability does not necessarily preclude justified choice, as long as the incommensurables in question are each rationally eligible to be chosen. Raz believes reasons can determine the rational eligibility of options, after which a person must simply determine the choice through an exercise of will. What justifies the choice of one rationally eligible alternative over another one is a person's bare act of choosing. We might call this form of justification a "performative justificatory act" wherein the stamp of a person's will gives the actual choice its moral legitimacy and authority. Returning to the case of Sartre's idealistic young man, his leaving to join the Free French Forces and his staying to care for his mother are each rationally eligible options. Ultimately, he must make a radical choice for one or the other. Whichever of these eligible options he chooses will be justified, for it is his performative act of willing that gives his choice its moral authority. Raz's solution, I think, is appealing. In everyday life, this seems to be our only way out of the incommensurability problem. When faced with incommensurable alternatives, such as whether to spend a year working and saving money or traveling to experience endangered ecosystems before their imminent collapse, or, to take an example pertinent to this chapter, whether to enroll in a Phase I trial to help advance scientific knowledge or to spend the next year visiting one's relatives, it seems to me that in such cases the heart decides and the mind rationalizes the decision. As long as our incommensurable options are each rationally eligible, that is, each reasonably worthy of choice, then we must simply put our will behind one of these options and accept responsibility for our choice. If this is correct, then justified choice is possible in the face of incommensurability and incomparability.

I believe Raz's solution comes, however, with two important caveats for our discussion of stem cell–based clinical trials. First, it is crucial for this approach that the deliberator actually makes a willful choice. Hypothetical choice or hypothetical choice scenarios are insufficient to justify the prioritization of one incommensurable option over another. This is because the final justification behind a choice comes directly from the deliberator's actually willing it. Second, along a related point, this willful choice must be made over an option that directly affects the deliberator. As I interpret it, Raz's willful choice solution to incommensurability is a variant of one's exercise of personal autonomy and thus the moral authority of one's willful choice derives from this aforementioned right to self-determination. Some observers may wonder whether such a radical, self-justifying choice is actually protected under the aegis of personal autonomy, because the deliberator cannot actually offer a reason for his choice; he can only acknowledge that he has willed the choice into action. Yet I believe, as I have written elsewhere, that a person's acting on a radical choice can be autonomous as long as the incommensurable value he chooses to pursue is authentic to him (Hyun 2001; 2002).

These two caveats have important implications for our discussion of stem cell–based clinical trials. The willful choice solution to the incommensurability problem rules out notion that researchers, regulators, and sponsors can simply sit in a room and determine amongst themselves what reasonable patient subjects are likely to want and then simply use this hypothetical choice to justify the risk-benefit ratio for a Phase I trial. Such an approach to resolving the incommensurability problem goes against the caveats outlined in the preceding text – that is, willful choice by a deliberator making a self-determining decision for himself. Not even a deliberative democratic procedure or some other means for achieving moral consensus within a group can adequately stand in as a substitute for Raz's willful choice solution, not unless (a) the deliberating group includes the full set of patient subjects who will actually enroll in the clinical trial and (b) there is unanimous agreement within this full set of actual research subjects, or alternatively, (c) there is some morally legitimate, politically modeled system of representation at work within the group such that actual patient research subjects do not have to be present during the deliberation but instead can have their "vote" represented by others authorized to make a willful choice on their behalf. Circumstances (a), (b), and (c) all seem to falter against the practical limitation that the actual research subjects in a clinical trial cannot be identified *ex ante* and consulted for the task of balancing the risk-benefit ratio prior to the subject recruitment period of the trial. Furthermore, circumstance (c) seems to take the political metaphor of representative democracy too far in trying to solve the philosophical moral problem of incommensurability. There is no analogous "political representation" for patient research subjects that would preserve the moral authority of personal autonomy undergirding Raz's willful choice solution. Given the disconnect in membership between the deliberating group and the future research subject group, not even the tools of sociological research (such as poll taking, focus groups, or qualitative in-depth interviews with patient populations) are up to the task of resolving the incommensurability of options during clinical trial design.

That said, it is clear to me that there is still an important role patients can play in the trial design phase of research. Patients and patient advocacy groups could help researchers and other trial administrators determine the range of rationally eligible options for potential research subjects. As I have argued in the previous section, the priorities and perspectives of patients are important for setting the design parameters of a clinical trial, especially in terms of defining the efficacy endpoints and judging the magnitudes of potential harms and benefits of the proposed therapy. As other authors have noted, there are no widely accepted standards for judging risk, benefit, and value in Phase I clinical trials (Anderson and Kimmelman 2010). Patients need to help set these standards of evaluation because ultimately it is for the betterment of patients that stem cell–based therapies are being proposed.

To summarize, I want to be clear that, by including patient viewpoints to help set the range of rationally eligible options, we do not thereby resolve the incommensurability problem. Rather, once a set of rationally eligible options has been deliberated upon and offered, it is up to individual research subjects to make a radical choice and, ultimately, through their act of willfully choosing, authorize their research participation in the face of incommensurable values. Only in this way can the incommensurability problem be resolved, on a case-by-case basis, by each individual for him- or herself.[24] Admittedly, this is an imperfect solution to the incommensurability problem, because it offers too little too late in the way of being able to justify any particular ordering of incommensurable eligible options during the process of clinical trial design.

My conclusions in this section may strike some as disconcerting. This is perhaps because I am proposing that there are significant limitations to what human reason can prescribe in the face of value incommensurability. Other authors have noted that Phase I clinical trials involve an element of tragic choice on the part of research participants due to the extreme uncertainties surrounding what the actual sacrifices will be (Solbakk and Zoloth 2011). I agree, but I think the better term here is not a *tragic choice*, for that implies a heavy-hearted, lose-lose decision, but rather a *radical and willful choice*, for this implies determination and hope. When patients are faced with the prospect of participating in a Phase I stem cell–based clinical trial, it is the heart that will ultimately decide. Given the existence of what may be an ineliminable, nonrational element to research consent, a motivation fueled perhaps by a strong dose of therapeutic hope, it is imperative that others guard against the possibility of patient exploitation. A patient's willful choice to be involved in what may be a lifelong commitment creates for researchers and clinical trial administrators a duty to follow through and monitor the health and well-being of their research subjects.

## Conclusion

Stem cell–based clinical trials involve manners of assessment quite unlike other types of human trials. Unlike, for example, criminal trials or competitive time trials, stem cell–based trials can incorporate the points of view of different vested parties during trial design and research administration, all without necessarily undermining the reliability of the final determination. Patient involvement during trial design may actually improve the ethical aspects of the resulting trial and perhaps even its scientific value.

---

[24] One of the philosophical consequences of my argument here is that it would be impossible for children and other decisionally incapacitated patients to resolve for themselves the incommensurability problem, because persons must have a deep appreciation of each rationally eligible option before making their willful choice. By contrast, most bioethicists and research regulators do not usually permit surrogate consent for invasive and risky nontherapeutic research on children or mentally compromised adults, so this particular philosophical consequence of my argument should not be too worrisome.

However, in advocating for more patient involvement in all steps of the research process, we must be careful not to slip into the mistake of believing that there are no lurking dangers. Earlier in this chapter I used the trial by ordeal metaphor to convey some important aspects of the patient's disease experience. Central to that message was my suggestion that therapeutic hope may be a strong motivator for patients volunteering in a clinical trial. Trials by ordeal were believed to be under divine control, and the judicial judgment relied on whether the subject survived the test. Today, stem cell–based clinical trials are believed to be under rational, scientific control; but because of the incommensurability problem, we can be uncertain about the actual degree of rational choice involved at the patient participation level. Ultimately, the subjects of both types of trials must proceed on the basis of a nonrational hope. This surrender to faith does not then mean that trial administrators can shrug off their own responsibility for the outcome. Testing new stem cell–based biologics may involve a lifetime burden for patient volunteers, thus others have a duty to monitor their safety for the long term. Patient involvement in these trials must be recognized and treated as an ongoing Herculean effort.

This last figure of speech is appropriate, because the word *trial* can also be used to signify a difficult experience or a laborious task. I believe comparing trials to a Herculean effort is fitting for another reason. The twelve labors of Hercules is a well-known series of tales involving the Greek hero's efforts to seek penance for his accidental deeds. The second labor of Hercules involved his having to slay the Lernaean Hydra, a nine-headed monster with surprising regenerative powers. According to one version of the legend, Athena gave Hercules a golden sword, which he used to cut off the Hydra's immortal head and hide it under a rock (Kerenyi 1978). Having slain the monster, Hercules saved some of the Hydra's toxic blood to poison his arrows for his other adventures. In due course – long after he completed his twelve labors and received his penance from Hera – Hercules died a painful death after his tunic was inadvertently tainted with some of the Hydra's blood. This classic myth should remind us that patients participating in stem cell–based clinical trials may – like the hero Hercules – remain vulnerable to unexpected and seriously harmful reactions years after their trials have formally ended. Thus the long-term health monitoring of research subjects is crucial. How to handle this responsibly and to whom this duty of beneficence belongs are among the most important questions facing the ethics of testing new stem cell–based biologics in patients.

# 8

# Still the Sky Is Blue

## *Stem Cell Tourism and Medical Innovation*

Now are the woods all black, but still the sky is blue.[1]

The quote by Proust opening this chapter aptly symbolizes the hope many brave patients maintain in the face of debilitating, progressive diseases. For them the woods are growing dark, but the blue sky beyond remains their focus and motivation. Unfortunately for many who are gravely ill, time is running out and they simply cannot wait for the day when new stem cell advancements may be approved to help ameliorate their suffering. For some patients with intractable medical conditions, the possibility of receiving a stem cell–based intervention now, outside the context of a clinical trial, may be an alluring prospect.

People's faith in the power of stem cells today has helped feed a phenomenon widely known as "stem cell tourism." Stem cell tourism is a worrying new form of medical travel driven by hope and pretense. Clinics around the world are offering unproven stem cell–based therapies to desperate patients for a wide array of medical conditions. Many of these stem cell clinics have come under attack by scientists, clinicians, and bioethicists on grounds that they exploit seriously ill patients and threaten legitimate progress in the stem cell field (Hyun et al. 2008).

These concerns are supported by strong empirical evidence. For example, an analysis of online advertisements for stem cell therapies reveals that many clinics worldwide overpromise the benefits of their purported treatments and grossly downplay or ignore their attendant risks (Lau et al. 2008). None of these clinics back up their claims with credible preclinical studies or other published scientific evidence, and none has volunteered any indication of independent and qualified peer review of

[1] Marcel Proust, *Remembrance of Things Past*, vol. 1 (1913/1982, 130).

the requisite scientific rationale or any evidence of safety and efficacy. Whether the motive is outright profiteering or a good-faith attempt to help needy patients (as may be the case in some clinics that operate within standard hospital systems in China and India), the risk to patients of physical harm and financial exploitation remains extremely high.[2]

One might conclude from all this that stem cell tourism – as the travel metaphor suggests – is teeming with medical tourist traps selling inauthentic representations of real medical treatment to unsuspecting consumers. But this is not simply another case of buyer beware. At stake is the potential for serious harm to vulnerable patients, many of whom may be too young to opt out of the proffered treatment. As a case in point, a group of Israeli physicians has reported of a child who developed tumors in his brain and spinal cord after being treated with a series of poorly defined fetal stem cell transplants administered at a Moscow stem cell clinic (Amariglio et al. 2009). Adverse outcomes such as this, especially in the current unregulated international environment, could threaten to undermine the public's trust in the stem cell field, as well as the health of patients hoping for a stem cell cure.

In light of these serious problems, many people may assert that the only responsible route to the clinic, scientifically and ethically, is through FDA-approved clinical trials processes. Conventional wisdom may dictate that, like pharmaceutical drugs and the use of other biological therapeutics, stem cell–based therapies must pass through a series of controlled studies before they can be justifiably sold to patients outside a clinical trials context.

But conventional wisdom always admits of exceptions. In this chapter, I draw attention to circumstances in which patients outside of clinical trials are likely to receive innovative stem cell–based interventions. These circumstances involve stem cell interventions not initially amenable to a clinical trials approach, expanded access to investigational stem cell products ("compassionate use"), and off-label uses of FDA-approved stem cell products. Each of these stem cell circumstances has an analogue in recent medical history, be it cardiac transplant, cancer therapy, or pediatric medicine. Each of these historical examples belies the assumption that clinical trials constitute the only route to the development of new therapies. If, as I shall argue, some room must inevitably be set aside for responsible attempts at innovative stem cell–based therapies, then

---

[2] Personal communication with Alok Srivastava, Head of the Department of Hematology, Christian Medical College, Vellore, India.

the question becomes how one best ought to regulate these exceptional cases. I conclude by proposing one such regulatory approach.

To help set up my analysis, I begin with a discussion of medical travel for unproven stem cell–based therapies. A closer look at the complexities of stem cell tourism reveals why we must ultimately confront the issue of innovative stem cell–based therapies. Unless we tackle this issue proactively, we will find it very difficult to discern the differences between problematic stem cell tourism and acceptable medical travel for innovative therapies, especially as stem cell research advances closer to the clinic. How do we allow room for responsible attempts at innovative therapies while sanctioning against problematic stem cell tourism? To answer this question, we must first examine the contours of the playing field between these opposing goal posts.

## The Complexities of Stem Cell Tourism

At present there exists broad international consensus that stem cell tourism is a serious problem. Although it would be tempting to condemn all stem cell tourism entirely, I believe our analysis of this phenomenon must go beyond simple and familiar concerns about consumer fraud, lack of scientific justification, and patient safety. The issues we need to address here can be far more nuanced than this, for they call into action our jumbled intuitions about medical travel more generally and the appropriate confines of medical innovation.

The topic of medical travel is quite complicated (Cohen 2011). Demonizing all stem cell tourism runs the risk of giving short shrift to patients' legitimate ethical motivations for such travel. Patients are not to blame, because medical travel may represent for them their last grasp of hope. Medical travel occurs in other areas of medicine, often involving highly innovative interventions at great cost to seriously ill patients, as happens today in cardiac centers of excellence all over the United States. Likewise, medical travel now and in the future may include "proven stem cell therapies" – that is, stem cell–based treatments that have been established in the clinic and accepted by the scientific and clinical community. Proven treatments like hematopoietic stem cell transplantation for leukemia may not be available to patients in their own country. In due course, other proven treatments may be banned in some areas for political or religious reasons because of their use of hES cells. Patients should remain free to travel to clinics offering established stem cell–based therapies. Thus we must be able to distinguish between acceptable medical travel for innovative, proven therapies and problematic stem cell tourism.

Thinking seriously about stem cell tourism will also require us to articulate the acceptable conditions under which unproven stem cell therapies may be offered to patients outside carefully controlled clinical trials. This will not be an easy task. The distinction between acceptable medical travel and problematic stem cell tourism cannot be based merely on the difference between proven and unproven therapies. Generally speaking, proven therapies are those that produce statistically significant health improvements that can be reasonably reproduced in similar patients. Unproven therapies are those that have not (yet) been shown to possess these two key elements. Despite this general distinction, it is not obvious that medical travel for unproven therapies is always ethically unacceptable. For example, medical travel occurs in other areas of medicine that also involve highly innovative and unproven interventions, such as face transplantation and conjoined twin separation, as occurs today in medical centers of excellence in the United States and abroad. The benefits of these interventions, when successful, can be tremendous. So, the bare conceptual distinction between proven and unproven therapies does not get us very far in understanding what makes medical travel for unproven stem cell therapies ethically problematic. In summary, the problem of stem cell tourism cannot reside per se in the unproven nature of the therapy or in the unfortunate reality that some patients may have to cross state or national borders for therapies that are otherwise unavailable at home.

## Innovative Therapies Are Grounded in Patient Care

I have suggested that the distance between problematic stem cell tourism and acceptable pursuits of innovative therapies may be far less than we might expect, with fewer markers in between to indicate their differences. Knowing what these differences are depends on how we answer the following set of questions. Under what circumstances should unproven stem cell–based innovations be allowed outside the context of a clinical trial? And how should attempts at innovative stem cell–based therapies be regulated? A few conceptual distinctions will help us frame our approach to answering these questions.

Stem cell tourism highlights the need for the regulation of innovative therapies. But what exactly would we be regulating, and what form should these regulations take? It is important to recall that, unlike

guidelines – which are unenforced general recommendations for professional conduct – regulations are a set of specific standards for which one
can be either in compliance or out of compliance, and for which there is
an enforcement mechanism in place to sanction against noncompliant
behavior (see Chapter 4). While guidelines and regulations are meant
to steer behavior at the local and individual level, regulations (because
of their greater specificity) are far less flexible and quickly adaptable to
sudden changes in the area in which they govern. Thus, in asking how
stem cell–based innovative therapies ought to be regulated, one needs to
recognize that there exists the potential for regulations to slow down the
rate of progress. Regulations are meant to harmonize practices and provide safeguards, and in that way they may promote advancements, but
there is no guarantee of these benefits if the regulations are not properly
calibrated to the dynamics of the area in question. In short, a regulatory
approach will have to be sensitive to the dynamics of the stem cell field.
We want to allow room for innovative therapies without condoning bad
practices.

Furthermore, guidelines and regulations cannot be created without
overarching rationales to justify their need. Regulations in particular
are meant to operationalize value commitments that have been made at
an abstract, theoretical level. In asking how stem cell–based innovative
therapies ought to be regulated, one must pause to consider the value
commitments motivating this question. Medically innovative therapies
are driven by a different set of goals than research, so it would be inappropriate to propose a set of regulations for innovative therapies that is
really aimed at promoting the goals of research. As the Belmont Report
spells out, research and innovative medical care serve different purposes.
Research aims to produce generalizable knowledge about new clinical
treatments. Notably, the individual patient's benefit is not the focus of
clinical research; neither is the individual patient's benefit the primary
focus of the human subjects research committees overseeing clinical
research (Agich 2001). In contrast, innovative therapies do not aim to
produce generalizable knowledge but are aimed primarily at providing
new forms of clinical care that have a reasonable chance of success for
individual patients with few or no acceptable medical alternatives. As the
Belmont Report explains, the mere fact that a procedure is medically
innovative does not qualify it as clinical research. Unlike research, the
main goal of innovative care is to improve or ameliorate an individual
patient's condition.

For the remainder of this discussion, then, the key point to keep in mind is that the regulation of stem cell–based innovative therapies must serve the purposes of good patient care. To argue against innovative stem cell–based care because it does not advance the goals of research (i.e., because it may not produce generalizable knowledge and the like) would be to misunderstand the value commitments that motivate medical innovation. The ethics of innovative therapies are at heart the ethics of proper patient care, not the ethics of clinical research, although there are similarities between the two spheres, mostly with respect to acceptable risk and voluntary informed consent. From many patients' point of view, however, consenting to medically innovative care may be preferable to enrolling in a clinical trial, especially where patient care is decidedly not the purpose of the trial – expanding knowledge is. Patients with precious little time might not care much about expanding knowledge; what they care about is getting better and surviving. Demonizing stem cell tourism will never squelch this vital instinct. Acceptable channels must be made available to seriously ill patients.

This is not to say that placing innovative stem cell–based therapies under the paradigm of good patient care automatically makes it less problematic ethically. The history of innovative therapies, particularly with respect to surgical innovations outside clinical trials, shows us that the outcomes for patients can often be tragic (Lombardo 2008). All innovative therapies are, by definition, risky and uncertain. The physician proposing an innovative therapy will normally lack the clinical equipoise (the epistemic and ethical neutrality over outcomes) necessary for conducting a clinical trial. That is, the physician must believe in her heart of hearts that the proposed therapy could benefit her patient. But due to her potential bias, she may not be the person best entrusted to obtain the patient's consent (Freedman 1987). And because of her lack of clinical equipoise, the physician also might not be in the best position to assess objectively the risk-benefit ratio of her proposed innovative therapy. Although rigorous informed consent and a realistic assessment of the risks are crucial in all patient care, the need to maintain high standards in these two areas is especially acute for innovative therapies.

In summary, a regulatory approach to permitting and overseeing the conduct of innovative stem cell–based therapies needs to be sensitive to the rapidly moving pace of stem cell science while remaining focused on the ethics of good patient care, not research. Next I discuss three circumstances under which patients are quite likely to receive innovative stem cell–based therapies outside of a clinical trials context, circumstances that will create new pressure for regulation. I conclude with a proposed regulatory approach that might help meet these challenges.

### Innovative Therapies Can Help Advance the Stem Cell Field

Many people may continue to insist that the only responsible way to develop stem cell–based therapies is through FDA-approved clinical trials processes. But this belief is built on a simplistic understanding of stem cell–based therapies (and, for that matter, of medical progress more generally). As we saw in Chapter 2, the concept of a "stem cell–based therapy" is not all of one piece. Within this concept exists a very wide spectrum of possible interventions for which some room for innovative therapies may prove to be essential.

In the not-too-distant future, interventions could involve multipotent stem cells used in novel ways, derivatives of hES cells, or derivatives of reprogrammed somatic cells, such as iPS cells. Furthermore, clinical researchers can use the patient's own cells (autologous transplantation); a donor's cells (allogeneic transplantation), which would require immune suppression; genetically modified cells; cells used in their site of origin (homologous transfer); or cells used outside of their site of origin (nonhomologous transfer). The transferred cells can be delivered systemically or transplanted directly into a specific site (with or without a bioengineered medical device seeded with cells). Variations in cell dosage, frequency of cell transfer, and the stage of the disease process in which the intervention is attempted also complicate what is already a dizzying array of possibilities.

It would be quite surprising if this enormous range of possible stem cell–based interventions could all fit conveniently into traditional clinical trials processes. As discussed in Chapter 7, the FDA clinical trials multiple phase system was developed largely for the testing of pharmaceutical drugs to assess safety and toxicity (Phase I), efficacy (Phase II), and comparative efficacy (Phase III). However, as I had argued at length, there are key differences between pills, on the one hand, and stem cells and their derivatives, on the other. Given the diversity of possible therapies and the biologically context-dependent nature of stem cell behavior, some stem cell–based interventions may prove to be amenable to a multistage clinical trials approach, while others may align more along a surgical or transplantation paradigm for which a clinical trials approach has historically proven to be quite difficult to utilize (Cosgrove 2008).

We must be prepared for the possibility that many stem cell–based interventions, like surgical interventions, might not be amenable to a rigid clinical trials approach. For example, in the last forty years less than 20 percent of all surgical interventions were developed through a clinical trials process, with some specialties such as cardiac transplant and laparoscopic surgery arising entirely without clinical trials (Cosgrove 2008). This historical pattern may also hold true for some stem cell interventions, particularly those with a very significant surgical component.

Furthermore, allowing room for innovative therapy may benefit other stem cell–based therapies that are amenable to a clinical trials process. In developing new stem cell–based therapies, much work may need to be done to optimize a procedure before formal clinical trials can be initiated. This early work may include further standardizing the procedure and learning exactly which types of patients stand to benefit from the proposed intervention. For example, if stem cell–based replacement therapies for Parkinson's disease are to become clinically competitive with other accepted treatment options, such as neurotransmitter drugs and DBS, then the transplantation procedure will have to be tailor-made as much as possible with each patient's brain. Furthermore, because Parkinson's disease is a multisystem neurodegenerative disorder, and given the heterogeneity of the patient population, individualized treatment strategies will have to include complex combinations of oral medication, DBS, and neural transplantation (Koch et al. 2009). As such, stem cell–based therapies for Parkinson's disease are likely to emerge as one among many tools in a combined arsenal of different possible interventions, with the battle plans drawn on a case-by-case basis over patient-specific topographies. It may be some time, after observational experience is gained within the context of innovative patient care, that formal clinical trials for stem cell–based therapies for complex conditions can be initiated.

As I argued in the previous section, all innovative therapies must be grounded in the ethics of patient care. Thus the primary motive for any intervention should be the best interests of the patient, with utmost attention paid to the risks he or she is likely to incur. With respect to stem cell–based therapies, the risks are high and largely unknown. Most troubling are those interventions that are the furthest removed from currently accepted hematopoietic stem cell therapies for diseases of the blood. Typically, these concerning interventions will involve heavily manipulated cells used outside of their normal niche environments. Therefore, along the continuum of possible clinical interventions, proposed therapies at the more complex end of the scale will require the closest scrutiny, for they will be the most unpredictable and risky. For example, allogeneic transplantation may necessitate the use of immunological suppression for quite extended periods of time, thus imposing further potential harms on the recipient. Nonhomologous use may result in the unpredictable behavior of transferred cells. For these reasons, preclinical studies for safety are important, despite their acknowledged limitations.

Considerations such as these dictate the need for independent, stem cell–specific peer review prior to the administration of an intervention. Recently, a model for protecting patients and promoting innovative therapies was proposed by the Society of University Surgeons, which is instructive for how one might proceed with the oversight of newly proposed stem cell–based interventions. According to the society's ethical guidelines for surgical innovation, clinicians must submit their proposals to a local surgical innovations committee, which, like an ethical research board at a university, is to provide appropriate review of the scientific rationale for the proposed intervention and the informed consent process, but all for the sake of good patient care, not research (Biffl et al. 2008). As I explain in the following text, a similar type of innovations committee, made up of domain experts with no vested interest in the proposed procedure, may work well to oversee and approve proposed innovative stem cell–based therapies. This would take the responsibility for informed consent and risk assessment and disclosure solely out of the treating physician's hands and add a layer of peer review that would otherwise be missing. Review by an innovations committee may help ensure that the patient's interests and his or her care are promoted as far as possible in the face of a proposed innovative stem cell–based therapy.

## Expanded Access and Off-Label Uses of Stem Cells

Some observers may object to my preceding analysis by arguing that a patient care paradigm is inapplicable in the case of most innovative stem cell–based therapies. Critics may argue that the FDA restricts the medical use of stem cells in the United States to those that are minimally manipulated in culture for less than forty-eight hours under nonproliferating conditions, and because most stem cell–based interventions are likely to utilize cells that are more than minimally manipulated, it appears that innovative physicians would not be allowed to use most stem cell products outside of a clinical trials context. Thus my concerns about the possibility of unregulated innovative stem cell–based therapies may seem irrelevant, at least in the United States.

This critique, however, overlooks some crucial facts.[3] Under current FDA policies, there are at least two ways in which physicians may administer more-than-minimally manipulated stem cell products and other biologics to patients. The first is under the FDA program for expanded access to investigational drugs and biological products for treatment use (what is sometimes referred to as "compassionate use"). The second is the off-label prescribing of FDA-approved stem cell products. A brief review of each of these routes reveals the need for an independent peer review process similar to the one outlined in order to ensure proper patient protections and care.

According to FDA policies made effective in late 2009, physicians may now request access to investigational drugs and biological products to treat individual patients and intermediate-size patient populations between ten and one hundred. According to the FDA, its revised rules for expanded access are intended to "improve access to investigational drugs for patients with serious or immediately life-threatening diseases or conditions who lack other therapeutic options and who may benefit from such therapies."[4] Physicians can request FDA permission to administer investigational biological products (such as more-than-minimally manipulated stem cells and their derivatives) as long as these products are being tested elsewhere in a clinical trial and only if expanded access will not interfere with the conduct of clinical investigations. In order to request expanded access for individual patients or intermediate-size patient populations, physicians must submit an application that includes the rationale for intended use, patient selection criteria, a description of the manufacturing facility and the method of administration to the patient, toxicology information, and assurance of IRB approval. In the case of individual patient use, the FDA is even willing to consider expanded access to investigational drugs and biological products for which there is "no relevant clinical experience" and for which "the

---

[3] This critique also assumes too narrow of a view. Interventions that are not FDA approved might still be offered overseas, and to shrug off any further discussion of stem cell–based innovative therapies based on current FDA standards would be to advance a U.S.-centric response to the international problem of stem cell tourism, much of which involves American patients traveling abroad. The question of whether and how to regulate stem cell–based innovative therapies is an issue for all countries, not just the United States.

[4] 21 C.F.R. § 312 and § 316 (2009), at 40900.

case for the potential benefit may be based on preclinical data or on the mechanism of action."[5]

The FDA revised expanded access program should be generally admired for clarifying some existing regulations and adding new types of expanded access for treatment use. Nevertheless, there is little reassurance provided in the FDA policies for those concerned about innovative stem cell–based therapies in the current environment of stem cell tourism. It is not difficult to imagine how stem cell clinics in the United States could offer new stem cell treatments to seriously ill patients, as long as their physicians gain permission through the expanded access program. Some stem cell clinics may learn to "game the system" by first subjecting complex stem cell products to the FDA clinical trials process for secondary indications that are less complicated and less expensive to investigate formally. Then they or others can request access to these novel stem cell biologics to treat patients outside of a clinical trial. Rather than helping to curb medical travel for unproven stem cell therapies, the FDA expanded access program may actually facilitate it within U.S. borders.

The FDA correctly acknowledges that expanded access is not research. It explains that expanded access use is "meant to diagnose, monitor, or treat a patient's disease or condition, not to generate scientific data intended to characterize the drug [or biological product]."[6] Interestingly however, the FDA requires IRB review of expanded access, even for individual patient use. Its stated rationale is that Congress intended the FDA to require IRB review consistent with the FDA responsibilities regarding treatment uses of investigational products.[7]

Whether one finds this rationale sufficient to justify an IRB approval requirement for expanded access, the key problem is that IRBs are not well suited to evaluate the scientific complexities of stem cell–based therapies. The chief purposes of an IRB are to evaluate informed consent procedures and risk-benefit ratios for research participation – not for the administration of innovative therapies. The goal of an IRB is to promote responsible research, not patient care or patient advocacy. (Recall that IRBs are supposed to weigh the risks to human research participants against the potential benefits to science and society – an ethical balancing act between two competing values that is normally not sanctioned in the context of medical care aimed at promoting a patient's best interests.)

---

[5]  Ibid., at 40912.
[6]  Ibid., at 40906, my brackets.
[7]  Ibid., at 40921.

Neither is there any assurance that the FDA is equipped to provide the necessary stem cell expertise or the focus on patient care that is essential for the evaluation of any proposed innovative stem cell–based therapy. An intermediary review system is therefore necessary, residing in the gap between the FDA, on the one hand, and individual physician judgment and IRB approval, on the other.

Off-label prescribing is another potentially troubling avenue through which patients in the future may receive unproven stem cell therapies. When a drug or biological product gains FDA approval for a particular use, physicians are free to use it in other populations for other indications, as long as they judge it to be of potential benefit. Off-label prescribing is premised on the position that the FDA does not have the authority to regulate medical practice and the assumption that physicians can be trusted to use their professional judgment in deciding how to treat their patients (Dresser and Frader 2009).

Historically, off-label prescribing has been an important boon for some specialties such as psychiatry, oncology, and pediatrics (as very few drugs have been tested specifically on children). Today, off-label use has become very widespread. As much as 21 percent of all prescribed medications are used for non-FDA-approved situations (Gillick 2009). And among all drugs prescribed off-label, 73 percent lacked evidence of clinical efficacy and only 27 percent had scientific evidence of efficacy (Radley et al. 2006). There is little reason to believe that FDA-approved stem cell products will be immune to current medical trends in off-label prescribing in the United States.[8] As soon as a complex stem cell product is approved by the FDA for one clinical use, it can be quickly snatched up as a tool for innovative stem cell–based therapies. According to current American medical professional norms, it is up to individual physicians to decide whether they will offer patients a stem cell therapy off-label.

The risk to patients posed by off-label prescribing has been discussed at a more general level by several commentators. Some have called for more government oversight and more stringent informed consent requirements so that patients are properly informed of the uncertainties of off-label uses (Dresser and Frader 2009). One group from the University of Pittsburgh School of Medicine and Pharmacy has recommended a procedure for reviewing off-label prescribing. This "in-house" policy includes an objective assessment of the quality of the supporting

---

[8] It bears mentioning that off-label prescribing is not typically permitted in the United Kingdom and in many European countries.

data for an off-label use, an explanation of the proposed intervention, multidisciplinary review, patient consent, and an assessment of safety and clinical outcomes (Ansami et al. 2006). A major advantage of this local peer review policy is that it may provide an added, flexible level of review that is well attuned to the goals of promoting patient care – an aim that IRBs are not meant to fulfill.

## Chartering a Way Forward

It is clear from the preceding discussions that a policy should be developed to protect patients and to foster responsible attempts at innovative therapies within the stem cell field. The possibility of innovative stem cell–based therapies cannot be ignored given current FDA policies and the nature of many conceivable stem cell therapies.

It should be noted, however, that the development of stem cell–based therapies through a medical innovations route alone is probably not desirable. One of the major advantages of a clinical trials approach is that it allows the results of a new procedure to be compared with the long-term outcomes of alternative interventions. This is especially important for stem cell–based therapies, because these are usually meant to be replacement therapies for which long-term survival, lasting efficacy, and lack of serious side effects are essential. Therefore, relying on medically innovative care alone will not do if we are interested in knowing how well stem cell–based therapies compare to other possible alternative interventions. Ideally then, the development of innovative stem cell–based therapies and the clinical trials process should work in a complementary manner.

Given the importance of clinical trials and medical innovation, how should the stem cell field proceed toward the clinic? The ISSCR *Guidelines for the Clinical Translation of Stem Cells* has attempted to address both of these avenues. First, the guidelines emphasize a clinical trials approach for the majority of cases involving the use of stem cells and their derivatives in patients (Hyun et al. 2008). As discussed in Chapter 7, fundamental principles in the ISSCR guidelines for the responsible administration of stem cell biologics in humans are (1) that only quality-controlled cells with known biological characteristics be used; (2) that efficacy and safety have been demonstrated in appropriate animal models whenever possible; (3) that stem cell–specific expertise is involved in the peer review of the clinical protocols and the underlying preclinical research; and (4) that voluntary informed consent is obtained prior to a clinical trial to ensure that recipients are aware of the risks of tumor formation and lack of proof of clinical benefits.

Crucial to our current discussion is the fact that the ISSCR guidelines also offer a set of stem cell–specific criteria for responsible attempts at medically innovative care in exceptional circumstances. Notably, these criteria can be used to distinguish problematic stem cell tourism from legitimate attempts at medical innovation. Both will involve "unproven" stem cell–based therapies, but there are crucial differences (Lindvall and Hyun 2009).

The first category of unproven therapy is that which is attempted without scientific rationale. Administering a stem cell–based intervention under these circumstances would be professionally and ethically irresponsible. It will not help the patient, the risks for adverse effects may be high, and it will not contribute to the development of clinically established stem cell therapies. Unfortunately, many stem tourism clinics today pay no heed to these concerns.

The second category of unproven stem cell–based therapy covers approaches that have a scientific rationale for which efficacy and lack of serious side effects may have been demonstrated in animal models, but the approach is not yet clinically established as safe and effective. This may be because the number of cells available for transplantation is severely limited, or because, as is the case of Parkinson's disease, further optimization of the procedure is necessary before a formal clinical trials process can be initiated. This category is identical to innovative therapies, which should be acceptable outside formal clinical trials in patients who lack good therapeutic options. Even stem cell–based innovative therapies should, however, be subject to scientific and ethical review and proper patient protections.

Thus the ISSCR guidelines for medical innovation are as follows. First there should be a written plan that includes (1) the scientific rationale; (2) any available evidence of efficacy and safety from preclinical studies in animal models as well as from applications of this intervention for other indications in humans; (3) the full characteristics of the cells to be delivered; (4) a description of the mode of cell delivery; and (5) a plan for the patient's clinical follow-up and care. This plan should be approved through a review process performed by experts, and there should then be a rigorous voluntary informed consent. (Patients must be told that the proposed intervention may have never been tried on humans before, and that there is no guarantee that it will help them. It may even worsen their condition.) Next, transparency of this review process and institutional accountability are also desirable and crucial for continued public support of the stem cell field. Following one's experience with the medically innovative procedure, physician-scientists should, whenever possible, initiate a clinical trials process.

Due to the complexity of stem cell–based approaches and their strong foundation on basic research, medical innovations should only be applied by clinicians who are experts in the field and with close links to stem cell laboratories. The recommendation here echoes the concept of "field strength" advanced by some writing in the liver transplantation field – namely, that the team performing the innovative procedure should have proven successes in relevantly similar procedures (Cronin et al. 2001). Like all other attempts at medical innovation, the administration of unproved stem cell–based therapies must always be bound by the standards of professional medical conduct and the patient-centered norms of professional medical ethics. Notably, the ISSCR guidelines for innovative stem cell–based therapies echo the basic oversight model for surgical innovations proposed by the Society of University Surgeons and the Pittsburgh group's internal policy for off-label drug use, although each of these three sets of policies were developed independently of one another.

Unfortunately, as guidelines, the ISSCR recommendations are essentially an unenforced code of professional conduct. What is needed, therefore, is a policy with regulatory bite. I propose that the regulation of innovative stem cell–based therapies ought to consist in a mandate for local innovations committee approval before novel interventions can be attempted. Local committee approval, when conducted by domain experts, has the distinct advantage of providing a regulatory structure that is flexible and sensitive to dynamic changes in the field.

## Conclusion

Given the current preliminary stages of clinical translational work in the stem cell field, patients should continue to be counseled against traveling for "innovative" stem cell therapies. If and when the time comes that advances in the stem cell field warrant novel attempts at stem cell–based interventions, these attempts should be conducted after a local medical innovations committee has determined that there is sufficient scientific rationale for attempting the intervention. The current phenomenon of stem cell tourism provides ample evidence of patients' willingness to subject themselves to risky and unproven therapies. Persons with stem cell–specific expertise should help ensure that they are presented with treatment choices that are well informed by the latest research. The regulatory approach recommended here, although not foolproof, is at least a good way to help guarantee that patients' health interests are attended to carefully.

The issues raised in this chapter apply not just to stem cell therapies but to all areas of medicine in which innovations play a key role in advancing clinical practices. It is crucial to acknowledge that medically innovative care will always track along just outside the envelope of accepted clinical practice. With respect to the stem cell field, new FDA-approved stem cell therapies will always provoke innovative adjustments in their use and application. As novel stem cell therapies enter clinical practice in the future, the question of permissible medical innovation at the periphery of stem cell medicine will remain inescapable. In the near future, however, there will be a need to articulate further the acceptable conditions under which unproven stem cell therapies for specific diseases may be attempted, as medical innovation, in patients outside of clinical trials. In a world already flattened by the Internet and easy global travel, this task will become increasingly difficult, especially as authoritative preclinical stem cell studies and legitimate clinical trials begin to offer promising results to the public. Thus the public's interest in stem cell tourism is likely to increase as stem cell science advances toward the clinic. We must be prepared for this new dawn. There is much work ahead for the international community of researchers, clinicians, patient advocates, and regulators.

# Epilogue

The caravan of stem cell science travels onward. In the prologue I suggested opposite interpretations were possible for what gives stem cell science its tremendous momentum around the world. On the one hand, stem cell research is driven by inquiries within the ongoing narrative of science, first launched by explorations into developmental and cell biology and genetics, and further enabled through advances in tissue cultivation. On the other hand, stem cell research is also driven by the exciting practical applications of basic scientific discoveries and the commercial and patient interests that soon follow. Readers should now see why both of these interpretations of the caravan metaphor are correct. Stem cell science is truly a caravan in the most figurative sense of the word, for it is suggestive of wide-eyed exploration, commercial gain, and the hope for a better life. As stem cell science proceeds into the future, important questions need to be asked about how its progress will affect the rights and interests of those involved in the research and those whose well-being may hinge on its results.

I have argued that the amazing plasticity of human cells, which stem cell science has barely begun to expand, offers us new powers and new uncertainties, just as all transformative technologies have done since the seventeenth century. Secular bioethics provides society with a means to bridle these new powers and to steer through these new uncertainties, but there are limitations. The dual language of secular bioethics – both the present tense of deontological rights and duties and the future tense of consequentialist moral priorities – may not yet have a complete moral grammar to deal with structural problems lingering in our ethical discourse. These issues involve the limits of people's autonomy rights and beneficent duties, the scope of morally relevant consequences, and the incommensurability of fundamental values.

I am aware that this book raises many more questions than it answers. But such is the nature of philosophy and bioethics and any other area of probing intellectual inquiry. As John Steinbeck and Ed Ricketts once wrote, "An answer is invariably the parent of a great family of new questions" (1941, 166). Secular bioethics, like stem cell research, is an evolving area of human activity. Those of us who have made it our life's work to pursue secular ethical inquiry will no doubt find progress in this area underdeveloped as compared to many other fields in the arts and sciences (Parfit 1984, 453–4). This is not bad news. For progress to occur, posing the right questions and refining how we ask them are crucially important.

That said, the task of addressing the ethical issues surrounding stem cell research should not be a job left solely for the bioethicist. I have suggested throughout this book that there are no bright line distinctions demarcating where the boundaries lie among stem cell science, bioethics, and patient interests. Dealing with the philosophical and practical elements of ethical stem cell research will have to involve constant interactions among each of these three major points of view.

Unfortunately, these parties seem to be journeying down separate paths hidden in a dense forest.[1] Researchers are on a journey of discovery and are under great pressure to contribute in a meaningful way to stem cell science. Patients are also on a journey, a deeply personal journey requiring every concentration on their next step forward. Bioethicists are on a journey of sentinel watchfulness, preoccupied with the sounds emanating from the obscured paths around them. Every once in a while they all meet in an open glade and gaze at one another just before plunging back down their respective trails. We must encourage each to seek out the others and to travel together in the same direction. If we can do that, then I have great confidence in bioethics and the future of stem cell research.

---

[1]  I owe this metaphor to Mary Baker, an accomplished patient advocate.

# References

Adamo, Luigi, Olaia Naveiras, Pamela L. Wenzel, Shannon McKinney-Freeman, et al. 2009. "Biomechanical Forces Promote Embryonic Haematopoiesis," *Nature* 459: 1131–5.

Agich, George J. 2001. "Ethics and Innovation in Medicine," *Journal of Medical Ethics* 27: 295–6.

Ahrlund-Richter, Lars, Michele De Luca, Daniel R. Marshak, Megan Munsie, Anna Veiga, and Mahendra Rao. 2009. "Isolation and Production of Cells Suitable for Human Therapy: Challenges Ahead," *Cell Stem Cell* 4: 20–6.

Allday, Erin. 2011. "Stem Cell Injection May Help Katie Sharify." *San Francisco Chronicle*. December 14.

Allen, Colin. 2010. "Animal Consciousness." In *Stanford Encyclopedia of Philosophy*, ed. Edward N. Zalta. Stanford, CA: CSLI Metaphysics Research Lab. Available at http://plato.stanford.edu/entries/consciousness-animal/#quest (accessed June 3, 2010).

Allen, Colin, and Marc Bekoff. 1997. *Species of Mind: The Philosophy and Biology of Cognitive Ethology*. Cambridge MA: MIT Press.

Amariglio, Ninette, Abraham Hirshberg, Bernd W. Scheithauer, Yoram Cohen, et al. 2009. "Donor-Derived Brain Tumor Following Neural Stem Cell Transplantation in an Ataxia Telangiectasia Patient," *PLoS Med.* 6. Available at http://www.plosmedicine.org/article/info:doi/10.1371/journal.pmed.1000029 (accessed January 11, 2010).

Anderson, James A., and Jonathan Kimmelman. 2010. "Extending Clinical Equipoise to Phase 1 Trials Involving Patients: Unresolved Problems," *Kennedy Institute of Ethics Journal* 20: 75–98.

Andrews, Kristin. 2011. "Animal Cognition." In *Stanford Encyclopedia of Philosophy*, ed. Edward N. Zalta. Stanford, CA: CSLI Metaphysics Research Lab. Available at http://plato.stanford.edu/entries/cognition-animal/ (accessed June 5, 2010).

Ansami, Nicole, Robert Branch, Bethany Fedutes-Henderson, Thomas Smitherman, et al. 2006. "Innovative Off-Label Medication Use," *American Journal of Medical Quality* 21: 246–54.

Appelbaum, Paul S., Loren H. Roth, and Charles Lidz. 1982. "The Therapeutic Misconception: Informed Consent in Psychiatric Research," *International Journal of Law and Psychiatry* 5: 319–29.

Appelbaum, Paul S., Loren H. Roth, Charles Lidz, P. Benson, et al. 1987. "False Hopes and Best Data: Consent to Research and the Therapeutic Misconception," *Hastings Center Report* 17: 20–4.

Aquinas, Thomas. 1274/1948. *Summa Theologiae.* New York: Benziger Bros.

Associated Press. 2007. "Bush Remarks on Stem Cell Research." June 20, 2007.

Barresi, John, and Chris Moore. 1996. "Intentional Relations and Social Understanding," *Behavioral and Brain Sciences* 19: 107–54.

Barrilleaux, Bonnie, and Paul S. Knoepfler. 2011. "Inducing iPSCs to Escape the Dish," *Cell Stem Cell* 9: 103–11.

Bartlett, Robert. 1986. *Trial by Fire and Water: The Medieval Juridical Ordeal.* New York: Oxford University Press.

Baylis, Françoise, and Andrew Fenton. 2007. "Chimera Research and Stem Cell Therapies for Human Neurodegenerative Disorders," *Cambridge Quarterly of Healthcare Ethics* 16: 195–208.

Behringer, Richard R. 2007. "Human-Animal Chimeras in Biomedical Research," *Cell Stem Cell* 1: 259–62.

Berg, Jessica, and Nicole Deming. 2011. "New Rules for Research with Human Participants?" *Hastings Center Report* 41: 10–11.

Berg, Paul, David Baltimore, Sydney Brenner, Richard O. Roblin III, et al. 1975. "Summary Statement of the Asilomar Conference on Recombinant DNA Molecules," *Proceedings of the National Academy of Sciences* 72: 1981–4.

Bianchi, Diana W., Gretchen K. Zickwolf, Gary J. Weil, Shelly Sylvester, et al. 1996. "Male Fetal Progenitor Cells Persist in Maternal Blood for as Long as 27 Years Postpartum," *Proceedings of the National Academy of Sciences* 93: 705–8.

Biffl, Walter L., David A. Spain, Angelique M. Reitsma, Rebecca M. Minter, et al. 2008. "Responsible Development and Application of Surgical Innovations: A Position Statement of the Society of University Surgeons," *Journal of the American College of Surgeons* 206: 1204–9.

Bonyhadi, M. L., and H. Kaneshima. 1997. "The SCID-hu Mouse: An in vivo Model for HIV-1 Infection in Humans," *Molecular Medicine Today* 3: 246–53.

Breitbach, Martin, Toktam Bostani, Wilhelm Roell, Ying Xia, et al. 2007. "Potential Risks of Bone Marrow Cell Transplantation into Infarcted Hearts," *Blood* 110: 1362–9.

Brons, Gabrielle M., Lucy E. Smithers, Matthew W. Trotter, Peter Rugg-Gunn, et al. 2007. "Derivation of Pluripotent Epiblast Stem Cells from Mammalian Embryos," *Nature* 448: 191–5.

Brustle, Oliver, Khalid Choudhary, Khalad Karram, Anita Huttner, et al. 1998. "Chimeric Brains Generated by Intraventricular Transplantation of Fetal Human Brain Cells into Embryonic Rats," *Nature Biotechnology* 16: 1040–4.

Call, Josep, and Michael Tomasello. 2008. "Does the Chimpanzee Have a Theory of Mind? 30 Years Later," *Trends in Cognitive Sciences* 12: 187–92.

Callahan, Daniel. 2003. "Bioethics." In *Encyclopedia of Bioethics*, 3rd ed., ed. Stephen G. Post. New York: Macmillan Press.

Camp, Elisabeth. 2009. "A Language of Baboon Thought?" In *Philosophy of Animal Minds*, ed. Robert Lurz. New York: Cambridge University Press.

Campbell, Joseph. 1991. *The Masks of God*, Vol. 4: *Creative Mythology*. New York: Penguin Books.

Candland, Douglas Keith. 1993. *Feral Children and Clever Animals: Reflections on Human Nature*. New York: Oxford University Press.

Carrel, Alexis, and Montrose Burrows. 1911. "Cultivation of Tissues in Vitro and Its Technique," *Journal of Experimental Medicine* 13: 387–96.

Catalina, Puri, Rosa Montes, Gertru Ligero, Laura Sanchez, et al. 2008. "Human ESCs Predisposition to Karyotypic Instability: Is a Matter of Culture Adaptation or Differential Vulnerability among hESC Lines Due to Inherent Properties?" *Molecular Cancer* 7: 76.

Caulfield, Timothy, and C. Rachul. 2011. "Science Spin: iPS Cell Research in the News," *Clinical Pharmacology and Therapeutics* 89: 644–6.

Chang, Ruth. 1997. "Introduction." In *Incommensurability, Incomparability, and Practical Reason*, ed. Ruth Chang. Cambridge, MA: Harvard University Press.

Chomsky, Noam. 1968. *Language and Mind*. New York: Harcourt, Brace and World.

1980. "Human Language and Other Semiotic Systems." In *Speaking of Apes: A Critical Anthology of Two-Way Communication with Man*, ed. T. A. Sebeok and J. Umiker-Sebeok. New York: Plenum Press.

Cohen, Cynthia B. 2007. *Renewing the Stuff of Life: Stem Cells, Ethics, and Public Policy*. New York: Oxford University Press.

Cohen, Glenn I. 2010. "Medical Tourism: The View from Ten Thousand Feet (Policy and Politics)," *Hastings Center Report* 40: 11.

Coleman, Carl H., Jerry A. Menikoff, Jesse A. Goldner, and Nancy N. Dubler. 2005. *The Ethics and Regulation of Research with Human Subjects*. San Francisco: The LexisNexis Group.

Cosgrove, Delos M. 2008. "Ethics in Surgical Innovation: Vigorous Discussion Will Foster Future Progress," *Cleveland Clinic Journal of Medicine* Supplement 6: S6.

Cowan, Chad A., Jocelyn Atienza, Douglas A. Melton, and Kevin Eggan. 2005. "Nuclear Reprogramming of Somatic Cells after Fusion with Human Embryonic Stem Cells," *Science* 309: 1369–73.

Crockin, Susan L. 2010. "A Legal Defenses for Compensating Research Egg Donors," *Cell Stem Cell* 6: 99–102.

Cronin, David C., J. Michael Millis, and Mark Siegler. 2001. "Transplantation of Liver Grafts from Living Donors into Adults – Too Much, Too Soon," *New England Journal of Medicine* 344: 1633–7.

Daley, George Q. 2010. "Stem Cells: Roadmap to the Clinic," *Journal of Clinical Investigation* 120: 8–10.

2011. "Imperfect Yet Striking," *Nature* 478: 40–1.

Daley, George Q., Lars Ahrlund-Richter, Jonathan M. Auerbach, Nissim Benvenisty, et al. 2007. "The ISSCR Guidelines for Human Embryonic Stem Cell Research," *Science* 315: 603–4.

Daniels, Norman. 1996. *Justice and Justification*. New York: Cambridge University Press.

Davidson, Donald. 1982. "Rational Animals," *Dialectica* 36: 317–28.

De Coppi, Paolo, Georg Bartsch Jr., M. Minhaj Siddiqui, Tao Xu, et al. 2007. "Isolation of Amniotic Stem Cell Lines with Potential for Therapy," *Nature Biotechnology* 25: 100–6.

Department of Health, Education and Welfare. 1979. *Report of the National Commission for the Protection of Human Subjects of Biomedical and Behavioral Research (The Belmont Report)*. 44 Fed. Reg. 23, 192.

Descartes, Rene. 1637/1998. *Discourse on the Method*, 3rd ed. Donald A. Cress, trans. Indianapolis, IN: Hackett Publishing Company.

Dickenson, Donna. 2008. *Body Shopping: The Economy Fuelled by Flesh and Blood*. Oxford: Oneworld Publications.

Dimos, John T., Kit T. Rodolfa, Kathy K. Niakan, Laurin M. Weisenthal, et al. 2008. "Induced Pluripotent Stem Cells Generated from Patients with ALS Can Be Differentiated into Motor Neurons," *Science* 321: 1218–21.

Dresser, Rebecca, and Joel Frader. 2009 "Off-Label Prescribing: A Call for Heightened Professional and Government Oversight," *Journal of Law, Medicine & Ethics* 37: 476–86.

Dworkin, Gerald. 1970. "Acting Freely," *Nous* 4: 367–83.

Dworkin, Ronald. 1978. *Taking Rights Seriously*. Cambridge, MA: Harvard University Press.

Easton, M. C. 1897/2006. *Illustrated Bible Dictionary*. New York: Cosimo Classics.

Eder, M. L., A. D. Yamokoski, P.W. Wittmann, and E. D. Kodish. 2007. "Improving Informed Consent: Suggestions from Parents of Children with Leukemia," *Pediatrics* 119: 849–59.

Egli, Dieter, Jacqueline Rosains, Garret Birkhoff, and Kevin Eggan. 2007. "Developmental Reprogramming after Chromosome Transfer into Mitotic Mouse Zygotes," *Nature* 447: 679–85.

Egli, Dieter, Alice E. Chen, Genevieve Saphier, Douglas Powers, et al. 2011. "Impracticality of Egg Donor Recruitment in the Absence of Compensation," *Cell Stem Cell* 9: 293–4.

Emanuel, Ezekiel J. 2004. "Ending Concerns about Undue Inducement," *Journal of Law, Medicine & Ethics* 32: 100–5.

Flax, Jonathan D., Sanjay Aurora, Chunhua Yang, Clemence Simonin, et al. 1998. "Engraftable Human Neural Stem Cells Respond to Development Cues, Replace Neurons, and Express Foreign Genes," *Nature Biotechnology* 16: 1033–9.

Foot, Philippa. 2001. *Natural Goodness*. Oxford: Oxford University Press.

Frank, Natasha Y., Tobias Schatton, and Markus H. Frank. 2010. "The Therapeutic Promise of the Cancer Stem Cell Concept," *Journal of Clinical Investigation* 120: 41–50.

Frankfurt, Harry. 1971. "Freedom of the Will and the Concept of a Person," *Journal of Philosophy* 68: 5–20.

Freed, Curt R., Paul E. Greene, Robert E. Breeze, Wei-Yann Tsai, et al. 2001. "Transplantation of Embryonic Dopamine Neurons for Severe Parkinson's Disease," *New England Journal of Medicine* 344: 710–19.

Freedman, Benjamin. 1987. "Equipoise and the Ethics of Clinical Research," *New England Journal of Medicine* 317: 141–5.

Gallup, Gordon G. 1970. "Chimpanzees: Self-Recognition," *Science* 167: 341–3.

Gallup, Gordon G., James R. Anderson, and Daniel J. Shillito. 2002. "The Mirror Test." In *The Cognitive Animal: Empirical and Theoretical Perspectives on Animal Cognition*, ed. Marc Bekoff, Colin Allen, and Gordon Burghardt. Cambridge, MA: MIT Press.

Gardner, Beatrix T., and R. Allen Gardner. 1971. "Two-Way Communication with an Infant Chimpanzee." In *Behavior of Nonhuman Primates*, ed. A. M. Schrier and F. Stollnitz. New York: Academic Press.

Garner, Richard L. 1896. *Apes and Monkeys*. London: Osgood and McIlvaine.

Gillick, Muriel R. 2009. "Controlling Off-Label Medication Use," *Annals of Internal Medicine* 150: 344–7.

Goldstein, Ronald S., Micha Drukker, Benjamin E. Reubinoff, and Nissim Benvenisty. 2002. "Integration and Differentiation of Human Embryonic Stem Cells Transplanted to the Chick Embryo," *Developmental Dynamics* 225: 80–6.

Greene, Mark, Kathryn Schill, Shoji Takahashi, Alison Bateman-House, et al. 2005. "Moral Issues in Human-Non-Human Primate Neural Grafting," *Science* 309: 385–6.

Griffin, James. 1997. "Incommensurability: What's the Problem?" In *Incommensurability, Incomparability, and Practical Reason*, ed. Ruth Chang. Cambridge, MA: Harvard University Press.

Gurdon, J. B., T. R. Elsdale, and M. Fischberg. 1958. "Sexually Mature Individuals of *Xenopus laevis* from the Transplantation of Single Somatic Nuclei," *Nature* 182: 64–5.

Habermas, Jürgen. 1987. *The Philosophical Discourse of Modernity*. Frederick Lawrence, trans. Cambridge: Cambridge University Press.

Halme, Dina G., and David A. Kessler. 2006. "FDA Regulation of Stem-Cell-Based Therapies," *New England Journal of Medicine* 355: 1730–5.

Hamilton, Edith. 1942/1998. *Mythology*. New York: Little, Brown, and Company.

Harrison, Ross. 1907. "Observations on the Living Developing Nerve Fiber," *Proceedings of the Society for Experimental Biology and Medicine* 4: 140–3.

Hasegawa, Kouichi, Jordan E. Pomeroy, and Martin F. Pera. 2010. "Current Technology for the Derivation of Pluripotent Stem Cell Lines From Human Embryos," *Cell Stem Cell* 6: 521–31.

Hauser, Marc D., Noam Chomsky, and W. Tecumseh Fitch. 2002. "The Faculty of Language: What Is It, Who Has It, and How Did It Evolve?" *Science* 298: 1569–79.

Hayes, Catherine. 1951. *The Ape in Our House*. New York: Harper.

Healy, Sue D., and Victoria Braithwaite. 2000. "Cognitive Ecology: A Field of Substance?" *Trends in Ecology and Evolution* 15: 22–6.

Hegel, G. W. F. 1821/1991. *Elements of the Philosophy of Right.* H. B. Nisbet, trans. Allen W. Wood, ed. Cambridge: Cambridge University Press.

Hoehn, Margaret, and Melvin Yahr. 1967. "Parkinsonism: Onset, Progression and Mortality." *Neurology* 17: 427–42.

Huang, Pengyu, Zhiying He, Shuyi Ji, Huawang Sun, et al. 2011. "Induction of Functional Hepatocyte-like Cells from Mouse Fibroblasts by Defined Factors," *Nature* 475: 386–9.

Hyun, Insoo. 2001. "Authentic Values and Individual Autonomy," *Journal of Value Inquiry* 35: 195–208.

 2002. "Waiver of Informed Consent, Cultural Sensitivity, and the Problem of Unjust Families and Traditions," *Hastings Center Report* 32: 14–22.

 2006a. "Magic Eggs and the Frontier of Stem Cell Science," *Hastings Center Report* 36: 16–19.

 2006b. "Fair Payment or Undue Inducement?" *Nature* 442: 629–30.

 2008. "Stem Cells from Skin Cells: The Ethical Questons," *Hastings Center Report* 38: 20–2.

 2010. "Allowing Room for Innovative Stem Cell–Based Therapies outside Clinical Trials: Ethical and Practical Challenges," *Journal of Law, Medicine & Ethics* 38: 277–85.

 2011a. "The Bioethics of iPS Cell-Based Drug Discovery," *Clinical Pharmacology and Therapeutics* 38: 646–7.

 2011b. "Moving Human SCNT Research Forward Ethically," *Cell Stem Cell* 9: 295–7.

Hyun, Insoo, and Kyu Won Jung. 2006. "Human Research Cloning, Embryos, and Embryo-Like Artifacts," *Hastings Center Report* 36: 34–41.

Hyun, Insoo, Wenlin Li, and Sheng Ding. 2010. "Scientific and Ethical Reasons Why iPS Cell Research Must Proceed with Human Embyonic Stem Cell Research," *Stanford Journal of Law, Science & Policy*, November 2010. Available at http://www.stanford.edu/group/sjlsp/cgi-bin/users_images/pdfs/61_Hyun%20Li%20Ding%20Final.pdf (accessed November 7, 2010).

Hyun, Insoo, Konrad Hochedlinger, Rudolf Jaenisch, and Shinya Yamanaka. 2007. "New Advances in iPS Cell Research Do Not Obviate the Need for Human Embryonic Stem Cells," *Cell Stem Cell* 1: 367–8.

Hyun, Insoo, Olle Lindvall, Lars Ahrlund-Richter, Elena Cattaneo, et al. 2008. "New ISSCR Guidelines Underscore Major Principles for Responsible Translational Stem Cell Research," *Cell Stem Cell* 3: 607–9.

Hyun, Insoo, Patrick Taylor, Giuseppe Testa, Bernard Dickens, et al. 2007. "Ethical Standards for Human-to-Animal Chimera Experiments in Stem Cell Research," *Cell Stem Cell* 1: 159–63.

Ieda, Masaki, Ji-Dong Fu, Paul Delgado-Olguin, Vasanth Vedantham, et al. 2010. *Cell* 142: 375–86.

Inoue, H., and Shinya Yamanaka. 2011. "The Use of Induced Pluripotent Stem Cells in Drug Development," *Clinical Pharmacology & Therapeutics* 89: 655–61.

Institute of Medicine. 2011. *Chimpanzees in Biomedical and Behavioral Research: Assessing the Necessity.* Washington, DC: The National Academies Press.

International Society for Stem Cell Research. 2006. *Guidelines for the Conduct of Human Embryonic Stem Cell Research.* Available at http://www.isscr.org/ GuidelinesforhESCResearch/2917.htm (accessed December 1, 2011).

    2008a. *Guidelines for the Clinical Translation of Stem Cells.* Available at http://www.isscr.org/GuidelinesforClinicalTranslation/2480.htm (accessed August 4, 2011).

    2008b. "Researchers Tout Need for All Forms of Stem Cell Research." September 3, 2008. Available at http://www.isscr.org/press_releases/all_ forms.html (accessed September 4, 2008).

James, Daylon, Scott A. Noggle, Tomasz Swigut, and Ali H. Brivanlou. 2006. "Contribution of Human Embryonic Stem Cells to Mouse Blastocysts," *Developmental Biology* 295: 90–102.

Jonsen, Albert R. 1998. *The Birth of Bioethics.* New York: Oxford University Press.

Jullien, Jerome, Vincent Pasque, Richard P. Halley-Stott, Kei Miyamoto, et al. 2011. "Mechanisms of Nuclear Reprogramming by Eggs and Oocytes: A Deterministic Process?" *Nature Reviews Molecular Cell Biology* 12: 453–9.

Kaitin, K. I. 2008. "Obstacles and Opportunities in New Drug Development," *Clinical Pharmacology & Therapeutics* 83: 210–12.

Kaminski, Juliane, Josep Call, and Michael Tomasello. 2008. "Chimpanzees Know What Others Know, But Not What They Believe," *Cognition* 109: 224–34.

Kant, Immanuel. 1785/1959. *Groundwork of the Metaphysics of Morals.* H. J. Paton, trans. London: Harper.

Karpowicz, Phillip, Cynthia B. Cohen, and Derek van der Kooy. 2004. "It Is Ethical to Transplant Human Stem Cells into Nonhuman Embryos," *Nature Medicine* 10: 331–5.

    2005. "Developing Human-Nonhuman Chimeras in Human Stem Cell Research: Ethical Issues and Boundaries," *Kennedy Institute of Ethics Journal* 15: 107–34.

Kass, Leon R. 2002. *Life, Liberty and the Defense of Dignity: The Challenge for Bioethics.* San Francisco: Encounter Books.

    2008. "Defending Life and Dignity." *Weekly Standard* 13. February 25, 2008.

Katsnelson, Alla. 2011. "Why Fake It? How 'Sham' Brain Surgery Could Be Killing Off Valuable Therapies for Parkinson's Disease," *Nature* 476: 143–4.

Kawai, Tatsuo, A. Benedict Cosimi, Thomas R. Spitzer, Nina Tolkoff-Rubin, et al. 2008. "HLA-Mismatched Renal Transplantation without Maintenance Immunosuppression," *New England Journal of Medicine* 358: 353–61.

Kellogg, W. N., and L. A. Kellogg. 1933. *The Ape and the Child: A Study of Environmental Influence upon Early Behavior.* New York: McGraw-Hill.

Kerenyi, Carl. 1978. *The Heroes of the Greeks.* H. L. Rose, trans. New York: Thames and Hudson.

Kerr, Douglas A., Jeronia Llado, Michael J. Shamblott, Nicholas J. Maragakis, et al. 2003. "Human Embryonic Germ Cell Derivatives Facilitate Motor Recovery of Rats with Diffuse Motor Neuron Injury," *Journal of Neuroscience* 23: 5131–40.

Kim, Dohoon, Chun-Hyung Kim, Jung-Il Moon JI, Young-Gie Chung, et al. 2009. "Generation of Human Induced Pluripotent Stem Cells by Direct Delivery of Reprogramming Proteins," *Cell Stem Cell* 4: 472–6.

Kim, K., A. Doi, B. Wen, K. Ng, et al. 2010. "Epigenetic Memory of Induced Pluripotent Stem Cells," *Nature* 467: 285–90.

Kim, Scott Y. H., Samuel Frank, Robert Holloway, Carol Zimmerman, et al. 2005. "Science and Ethics of Sham Surgery: A Survey of Parkinson Disease Clinical Researchers," *Archives of Neurology* 62: 1357–60.

Kiskinis, Evangelos, and Kevin Eggan. 2010. "Progress toward the Clinical Application of Patient-Specific Pluripotent Stem Cells," *Journal of Clinical Investigation* 120: 51–9.

Klitzman, Robert, and Mark V. Sauer. 2009. "Payment of Egg Donors in Stem Cell Research in the USA," *Reproductive BioMedicine Online* 18: 603–8.

Koch, Philipp, Zaal Kokaia, Olle Lindvall, and Oliver Brustle. 2009. "Emerging Concepts in Neural Stem Cell Research: Autologous Repair and Cell-Based Disease Modelling," *Lancet Neurology* 8: 819–29.

Kola, Ismail, and John Landis. 2004. "Can the Pharmaceutical Industry Reduce Attrition Rates?" *Nature Reviews Drug Discovery* 3: 711–15.

Lakoff, George, and Mark Johnson. 1999. *Philosophy in the Flesh: The Embodied Mind and Its Challenge to Western Thought.* New York: Basic Books.

Landecker, Hannah. 2007. *Culturing Life: How Cells Became Technologies.* Cambridge, MA: Harvard University Press.

Lau, Darren, Ubaka Ogbogu, Benjamin Taylor, Tania Stafinski, et al. 2008. "Stem Cell Clinics Online: The Direct-to-Consumer Portrayal of Stem Cell Medicine," *Cell Stem Cell* 3: 591–4.

Laustriat, D., J. Gide, and M. Peschanski. 2010. "Human Pluripotent Stem Cells in Drug Discovery and Predictive Toxicology," *Biochemical Society Transactions* 38: 1051–7.

Lensch, M. William, Thorsten M. Schlaeger, Leonard I. Zon, and George Q. Daley. 2007. "Teratoma Formation Assays with Human Embryonic Stem Cells: A Rationale for One Type of Human-Animal Chimera," *Cell Stem Cell* 1: 253–8.

Lévi-Strauss, Claude. 1963. *Structural Anthropology,* Vol. 2. Claire Jacobson and Brooke Grundfest Schoepf, trans. New York: Basic Books.

Lewis, David. 1983. "Extrinsic Properties," *Philosophical Studies* 44: 197–200.

Li, Han, Manuel Collado, Aranzazu Villasante, Katerina Strati, et al. 2009. "The Ink4/Arf Locus Is a Barrier for iPS Cell Reprogramming," *Nature* 460: 1136–9.

Lindvall, Olle, and Insoo Hyun. 2009. "Medical Innovation versus Stem Cell Tourism," *Science* 324: 1664–5.

Lindvall, Olle, and Zaal Kokaia. 2010. "Stem Cells in Human Neurodegenerative Disorders – Time for Clinical Translation?" *Journal of Clinical Investigation* 120: 29–40.

Lindvall, Olle, Zaal Kokaia, and A. Martinez-Serrano. 2004. "Stem Cell Therapy for Human Neurodegenerative Disorders – How to Make It Work," *Nature Medicine* Supplement 10: S42–50.

Locke, John. 1690/1980. *Second Treatise of Government.* Indianapolis, IN: Hackett Publishing Company.

Lombardo, P. A. 2008. "A Historical Perspective: The More Things Change, the More They Remain the Same," *Cleveland Clinic Journal of Medicine* Supplement 6: S65–6.

Ma, Yilong, Chengke Tang, Thomas Chaly, Paul Greene, et al. 2010. "Dopamine Cell Implantation in Parkinson's Disease: Long-Term Clinical and [18]F-FDOPA PET Outcomes," *The Journal of Nuclear Medicine* 51: 7–15.

Macklin, Ruth. 1999. "The Ethical Problems with Sham Surgery in Clinical Research," *New England Journal of Medicine* 341: 992–6.

Maekawa, Momoko, Kei Yamaguchi, Tomonori Nakemura, Ran Shibukawa, et al. 2011. "Direct Reprogramming of Somatic Cells Is Promoted by Maternal Transcription Factor Glis1," *Nature* 474: 225–9.

Magnus, Tim, Ying Liu, Graham C. Parker, and Mahendra S. Rao. 2008. "Stem Cell Myths," *Philosophical Transactions of the Royal Society B: Biological Sciences* 363: 9–22.

Maherali, Nimet, Rupa Sridharan, Wei Xie, Jochen Utikal, et al. 2007. "Directly Reprogrammed Fibroblasts Show Global Epigenetic Remodeling and Widespread Tissue Contribution," *Cell Stem Cell* 1: 55–70.

Maitra, Anirban, Dan E. Arking, Narayan Shivapurkar, Morna Ikeda, et al. 2005. "Genomic Alterations in Cultured Human Embryonic Stem Cells," *Nature Genetics* 37: 1099–103.

Marx, Karl. 1845/1978. "The German Ideology." In *The Marx-Engels Reader*, 2nd ed., ed. Robert C. Tucker. New York: Norton and Company.

Mauro, Alexander. 1961. "Satellite Cell of Skeletal Muscle Fibers," *Journal of Biophysical and Biochemical Cytology* 9: 493–5.

Miles, H. Lyn. 1983. "Apes and Language: The Search for Communicative Competence." In *Language in Primates: Perspectives and Implications*, ed. Judith de Luce and Hugh T. Wildner. New York: Springer-Verlag.

Mill, John Stuart. 1859/1988. *On Liberty*. Indianapolis, IN: Hackett Publishing Company.
  1869/1988. *The Subjection of Women*. Indianapolis, IN: Hackett Publishing Company.

Millgram, Elijah. 1997. "Incommensurability and Practical Reasoning." In *Incommensurability, Incomparability, and Practical Reason*, ed. Ruth Chang. Cambridge, MA: Harvard University Press.

Mills, T. Wesley. 1898. *The Nature and Development of Animal Intelligence*. New York: Macmillan.

Mueller, Dawn, Michael J. Shamblott, Harold E. Fox, John D. Gearhart, et al. 2005. "Transplanted Human Embryonic Germ Cell-Derived Neural Stem Cells Replace Neurons and Oligodendrocytes in the Forebrain of Neonatal Mice with Excitotoxic Brain Damage," *Journal of Neuroscience Research* 82: 592–608.

Muotri, Alysson R., Kinichi Nakashima, Nicolas Toni, Vladislav M. Sandler, et al. 2005. "Development of Functional Human Embryonic Stem Cell–Derived Neurons in Mouse Brain," *Proceedings of the National Academy of Sciences* 102: 18644–8.

Najm, Fadi J., Josh G. Chenowerth, Philip D. Anderson, Joseph H. Nadeau, et al. 2011. "Isolation of Epiblast Stem Cells from Preimplantation Mouse Embryos," *Cell Stem Cell* 8: 318–25.

Nasr, Seyyed Hossein. 2002. *The Heart of Islam: Enduring Values for Humanity*. New York: Harper Collins.

National Academy of Sciences. 2005. *Guidelines for Human Embryonic Stem Cell Research*. Washington, DC: The National Academies Press.

National Research Council. 1996. *Guide for the Care and Use of Laboratory Animals*. Washington, DC: National Academies Press.

Nistor, Gabriel I., Minodora O. Totoiu, Nadia Haque, Melissa K. Carpenter, et al. 2005. "Human Embryonic Stem Cells Differentiate into Oligodendrocytes in High Purity and Myelinate after Spinal Cord Transplantation," *Glia* 49: 385–96.

Noggle, Scott, Ho-Lim Fung, Athurva Gore, Hector Martinez, et al. 2011. "Human Oocytes Reprogram Somatic Cells to a Pluripotent State," *Nature* 478: 70–5.

North, Trista E., Wolfram Goessling, Marian Peeters, Pulin Li, et al. 2009. "Hematopoietic Stem Cell Development Is Dependent on Blood Flow," *Cell* 137: 736–48.

Nuremberg Code. 1946–9. "Permissible Medical Experiments." In *Trials of War Criminals before the Nuernberg Military Tribunals under Control Council Law No. 10*, Vol. 2. Washington, DC: U.S. Government Printing Office, 181–4.

Okita, Keisuke, Tomoko Ichisak, and Shinya Yamanaka. 2007. "Generation of Germline-Competent Induced Pluripotent Stem Cells," *Nature* 448: 313–17.

Okita Keisuke, Masato Nakagawa, Hong Hyenjong, Tomoko Ichisaka, et al. 2008. "Generation of Mouse Induced Pluripotent Stem Cells without Viral Vectors," *Science* 322: 949–53.

Olanow, C. Warren, Christopher G. Goetz, Jeffrey H. Kordower, A. Jon Stoessl, et al. 2003. "A Double-Blind Controlled Trial of Bilateral Fetal Nigral Transplantation in Parkinson's Disease," *Annals of Neurology* 54: 403–14.

Orlans, F. B. 1993. *In the Name of Science: Issues in Responsible Animal Experimentation*. New York: Oxford University Press.

Ourednik, Vaclav, Jitka Ourednik, Jonathan D. Flax, W. Michael Zawada, et al. 2001. "Segregation of Human Neural Stem Cells in the Developing Primate Forebrain," *Science* 293: 1820–4.

Paludan, Ann. 1981. *The Imperial Ming Tombs*. New Haven, CT: Yale University Press.

Pang, Zhiping P., Nan Yang, Thomas Vierbuchen, Austin Ostermeier, et al. 2011. "Induction of Human Neuronal Cells by Defined Transcription Factors," *Nature* 476: 220–3.

Parfit, Derek. 1984. *Reasons and Persons*. Oxford: Oxford University Press.

Park, In-Hyun, Natasha Arora, Hongguang Huo, Nimet Maherali, et al. 2008. "Disease-Specific Induced Pluripotent Stem Cells," *Cell* 134: 877–86.

Park, In-Hyun, Rui Zhao, Jason A. West, Akiko Yabuuchi, et al. 2007. "Reprogramming of Human Somatic Cells to Pluripotency with Defined Factors," *Nature* 451: 141–6.

Patterson, Francine. 1978. "The Gestures of a Gorilla: Language Acquisition in Another Pongid," *Brain and Language* 5: 72–97.

Peerani, Raheem and Peter W. Zandstra. 2010. "Enabling Stem Cell Therapies through Synthetic Stem Cell–Niche Engineering," *Journal of Clinical Investigation* 120: 60–70.

Pentz, Rebecca D., Margaret White, R. Donald Harvey, Zachary Luke Farmer, et al. 2012. "Therapeutic Misconception, Misestimation, and Optimism in Participants Enrolled in Phase 1 Trials," *Cancer* 118: 4571–8.

Piccini, Paola, David J. Brooks, Anders Bjorklund, Roger N. Gunn, et al. 1999. "Dopamine Release from Nigral Transplants Visualized *in vivo* in a Parkinson's Patient," *Nature Neuroscience* 12: 1137–40.

Pinker, Steven. 1994. *The Language Instinct: How the Mind Creates Language.* New York: W. Morrow and Co.

Pollack, Andrew. 2011. "Geron Is Shutting Down Its Stem Cell Clinical Trial." *The New York Times.* November 14.

Polo, Jose M., Susanna Liu, Maria Eugenia Figueroa, Warakorn Kulalert, et al. 2010. "Cell Type of Origin Influences the Molecular and Functional Properties of Mouse Induced Pluripotent Stem Cells," *Nature Biotechnology* 28: 848–55.

Premack, David, and Ann James Premack. 1983. *The Mind of an Ape.* New York: Norton.

Premack, David, and Guy Woodruff. 1978. "Does the Chimpanzee Have a Theory of Mind?" *Behavioral and Brain Sciences* 1: 515–26.

Proust, Marcel. 1913/1982. *Remembrance of Things Past,* Vol. I. New York: Vintage.

Radley, David C., Stan N. Finkelstein, and Randall S. Stafford. 2006. "Off-Label Prescribing among Office-Based Physicians," *Archives of Internal Medicine* 166: 1021–6.

Rawls, John. 1971. *A Theory of Justice.* Cambridge, MA: Harvard University Press.

Raz, Joseph. 1986. *The Morality of Freedom.* Oxford: Oxford University Press.

1997. "Incommensurability and Agency." In *Incommensurability, Incomparability, and Practical Reason,* ed. Ruth Chang. Cambridge, MA: Harvard University Press.

Research!America. 2010. America Speaks, Poll Data Summary Volume 11. Available at http://www.researchamerica.org/uploads/AmericaSpeaksV11.pdf (accessed December 18, 2010).

Robert, Jason Scott, and Francoise Baylis. 2003. "Crossing Species Boundaries," *American Journal of Bioethics* 3: 1–13.

Robertson, John. 1978. "The Scientist's Right to Research: A Constitutional Analysis," *Southern California Law Review* 51: 1203.

Rollin, B. E., and M. L. Kesel. 1990. *The Experimental Animal in Biomedical Research.* Boston: CRC Press.

Rothman, David J. 1991. *Strangers at the Bedside: A History of How Law and Bioethics Transformed Medical Decision Making.* New York: Basic Books.

Rousseau, Jean-Jacques. 1754/1964. "Discourse on the Origin and Foundations of Inequality among Men." In *The First and Second Discourses.* ed. Roger D. Masters and trans. Judith R. Masters. New York: St. Martin's Press.

Roxland, Beth E. 2012. "New York State's Landmark Policies on Oversight and Compensation for Egg Donation to Stem Cell Research," *Regenerative Medicine* 7: 397–408.

Russell, Bertrand. 1945. *A History of Western Philosophy*. New York: Simon and Schuster.

Sartre, Jean-Paul. 1946/1975. "Existentialism Is a Humanism." In *Existentialism from Dostoevsky to Sartre*, ed. Walter Kaufman. New York: Meridian.

Satake, Wataru, Yuko Nakabayashi, Ikuko Mizuta, Yushi Hirota, et al. 2009. "Genome-Wide Association Study Identifies Common Varients at Four Loci as Genetic Risk Factors for Parkinson's Disease," *Nature Genetics* 41: 1303–7.

Sato, Noboru, Ignacio M. Sanjuan, Michael Heke, Makiko Uchida, et al. 2003. "Molecular Signature of Human Embryonic Stem Cells and Its Comparison with the Mouse," *Developmental Biology* 260: 404–13.

Schedl, Andreas, Allyson Ross, Muriel Lee, Dieter Engelkamp, et al. 1996. "Influence of PAX6 Gene Dosage on Development: Overexpression Causes Severe Eye Abnormalities," *Cell* 86: 71–82.

Schulman, Adam. 2008. "Bioethics and the Question of Human Dignity." In *Human Dignity and Bioethics: Essays Commissioned by the President's Council on Bioethics*. Washington, DC. Available at www.bioethics.gov (accessed February 20, 2010).

Schwartz, Steven D., Jean-Pierre Hubschman, Gad Heilwell, Valentina Franco-Cardenas, et al. 2012. "Embryonic Stem Cell Trials for Macular Degeneration: A Preliminary Report," *The Lancet* 379: 713–20.

Shapiro, Lawrence A. 2011. *Embodied Cognition*. New York: Routledge.

Shettleworth, Sara J. 2010. "Clever Animals and Killjoy Explanations in Comparative Psychology," *Trends in Cognitive Sciences* 14: 477–81.

Shreeve, Jamie. 2005. "The Other Stem Cell Debate." *New York Times Magazine*. Available at http://www.nytimes.com/2005/04/10/magazine/10CHIMERA.html (accessed April 10, 2005).

Shumaker, Robert W., and Karyl B. Swartz. 2002. "When Traditional Methodologies Fail: Cognitive Studies of Great Apes." In *The Cognitive Animal: Empirical and Theoretical Perspectives on Animal Cognition*, ed. Marc Bekoff, Colin Allen, and Gordon Burghardt. Cambridge, MA: MIT Press.

Skloot, Rebecca. 2010. *The Immortal Life of Henrietta Lacks*. New York: Crown Publishing Group.

Smart, Nicola, Sveva Bollini, Karina N. Dube, Joaquim M. Vieira, et al. 2011. "De Novo Cardiomyocytes from within the Activated Adult Heart after Injury," *Nature* 474: 640–4.

Solbakk, Jan Helge. 2011. "Persons versus Things," *Nature* 478: 41.

Solbakk, Jan Helge, and Laurie Zoloth. 2011. "The Tragedy of Translation: The Case of 'First Use' in Human Embryonic Stem Cell Research," *Cell Stem Cell* 8: 479–81.

Sollano, J. A., J. M. Kirsch, M. V. Bala, M. G. Chambers, and L. H. Harpole. 2008. "The Economics of Drug Discovery and the Ultimate Valuation of Pharmacotherapies in the Marketplace," *Clinical Pharmacology & Therapeutics* 84: 263–6.

Stadtfeld, Matthias, Masaki Nagaya, Jochen Utikal, Gordon Weir, et al. 2008. "Induced Pluripotent Stem Cells Generated without Viral Integration," *Science* 322: 945–9.

Stein, R. S., H. Brody, T. Tomlinson, D. M. Shaner, et al. "CPR-Not-Indicated and Futility," *Annals of Internal Medicine* 124: 75–7.

Stein, Rob. 2011. "Stem Cells Were God's Will, Says First Recipient of Treatment." *The Washington Post.* April 15.

Steinbeck, John, and Edward F. Ricketts. 1941. *Sea of Cortez: A Leisurely Journal of Travel and Research.* New York: Viking Press.

Stocker, Michael. 1997. "Abstract and Concrete Value: Plurality, Conflict, and Maximization." In *Incommensurability, Incomparability, and Practical Reason,* ed. Ruth Chang. Cambridge, MA: Harvard University Press.

Streiffer, Robert. 2005. "At the Edge of Humanity: Human Stem Cells, Chimeras, and Moral Status," *Kennedy Institute of Ethics Journal* 15: 347–70.

Szabo, Eva, Shravanti Rampalli, Ruth M. Risueno, Angelique Schnerch, et al. 2010. "Direct Conversion of Human Fibroblasts to Multilineage Blood Progenitors," *Nature* 468: 521–6.

Tabar, Viviane, Georgia Panagiotakos, Edward D. Greenberg, Bill K. Chan, et al. 2005. "Migration and Differentiation of Neural Precursors Derived from Human Embryonic Stem Cells in the Rat Brain," *Nature Biotechnology* 23: 601–6.

Takahashi Kazutoshi, and Shinya Yamanaka. 2006. "Induction of Pluripotent Stem Cells from Mouse Embryonic and Adult Fibroblast Cultures by Defined Factors," *Cell* 126: 663–76.

Takahashi Kazutoshi, Koji Tanabe, Mari Ohnuki, Megumi Narita, et al. 2007. "Induction of Pluripotent Stem Cells from Adult Human Fibroblasts by Defined Factors," *Cell* 131: 861–72.

Tedesco, Francesco Saverio, Arianna Dellavalle, Jordi Diaz-Manera, Graziella Messina, and Giulio Cossu. 2010. "Repairing Skeletal Muscle: Regenerative Potential of Skeletal Muscle Stem Cells," *Journal of Clinical Investigation* 120: 11–19.

Terrace, Herbert S. 1979. *Nim.* New York: Alfred A Knopf.

Terrace, Herbert S., Laura-Ann Petitto, R. J. Sanders, and T. G. Bever. 1979. "Can an Ape Create a Sentence?" *Science* 206: 891–902.

Tesar, Paul J., Josh G. Chenoweth, Francis A. Brook, Timothy J. Davies, et al. 2007. "New Cell Lines from Mouse Epiblast Share Defining Features with Human Embryonic Stem Cells," *Nature* 448: 196–9.

Testa, Giuseppe. 2009. "What to Do with the Grail Now That We Have It? iPSCs, Potentiality, and Public Policy," *Cell Stem Cell* 5: 358–9.

Thomas, E. Donnall. 1999. "A History of Haemopoietic Cell Transplantation," *British Journal of Haematology* 105: 330–9.

Thomas, E. Donnall, Harry L. Lochte Jr., Wan Ching Lu, and Joseph W. Ferrebee. 1957. "Intravenous Infusion of Bone Marrow in Patients Receiving Radiation and Chemotherapy," *New England Journal of Medicine* 257: 491–6.

Thomson, James A., Joseph Itskovitz-Eldor, Sander S. Shapiro, Michelle A. Waknitz, et al. 1998. "Embryonic Stem Cell Lines Derived from Human Blastocysts," *Science* 282: 1145–7.

Thorndike, Edward L. 1898. "Animal Intelligence: An Experimental Study of the Associative Processes in Animals," *Psychological Review, Monograph Supplement* 8: 1–109.

Varmus, Harold. 1999. "NIH Director's Statement on Research Using Stem Cells – 1/26/99," *Stem Cell Information: The National Institutes of Health Resource for Stem Cell Research*. Available at http://stemcells.nih.gov/policy/statements/statement.asp (accessed February 1, 1999).

Vierbuchen, Thomas, Austin Ostermeier, Zhiping P. Pang, Yuko Kokubu, et al. 2010. "Direct Conversion of Fibroblasts to Functional Neurons by Defined Factors," *Nature* 463: 1035–41.

von Uexküll, Jacob. 1934. *A Stroll through the Worlds of Animals and Men*. Berlin: Springer.

Wadman, Meredith. 2011. "Chimpanzee Research on Trial," *Nature* 474: 268–71.

Warnock, Mary. 1985. *A Question of Life: The Warnock Report on Human Fertilisation & Embryology*. Oxford: Basil Blackwell.

Warren, Luigi, Philip D. Manos, Tim Ahfeldt, Yuin-Han Loh, et al. 2010. "Highly Efficient Reprogramming to Pluripotency and Directed Differentiation of Human Cells with Synthetic Modified mRNA," *Cell Stem Cell* 7: 618–30.

Watson, Gary. 1975. "Free Agency," *Journal of Philosophy* 72: 205–20.

Weigel, George. 2005. *Witness to Hope: The Biography of Pope John Paul II*. New York: Harper Perennial.

Wernig, Marius, Alexander Meissner, Ruth Foreman, Tobias Brambrink, et al. 2007. "In Vitro Reprogramming of Fibroblasts into a Pluripotent ES-Cell-Like State," *Nature* 448: 318–24.

Westfall, Richard. 1999. *The Construction of Modern Science: Mechanisms and Mechanics*. Cambridge: Cambridge University Press.

Wiggins, David. 1997. "Incommensurability: Four Proposals." In *Incommensurability, Incomparability, and Practical Reason*, ed. Ruth Chang. Cambridge, MA: Harvard University Press.

Williams, Bernard. 1973. "A Critique of Utilitarianism." In *Utilitarianism: For and Against*, ed. J. J. C. Smart and Bernard Williams. Cambridge: Cambridge University Press.

Wilmut, Ian, A. E. Schnieke, J. McWhir, A. J. Kind, et al. 1997. "Viable Offspring Derived from Fetal and Adult Mammalian Cells," *Nature* 385: 810–13.

Wilson, Robert A., and Lucia Foglia. 2011. "Embodied Cognition." In *Stanford Encyclopedia of Philosophy*, ed. Edward N. Zalta. Stanford, CA: CSLI Metaphysics Research Lab. Available at http://plato.stanford.edu/entries/embodied-cognition/ (accessed June 5, 2010).

Wimmer, Heinz, and Josef Perner. 1983. "Beliefs about Beliefs: Representation and Constraining Function of Wrong Beliefs in Young Children's Understanding of Deception," *Cognition* 13: 103–28.

Witmer, Lightner. 1909. "A Monkey with a Mind," *Psychological Clinic* 3: 179–205.

Wood, Allen W. 2002. *Unsettling Obligations: Essays on Reason, Reality and the Ethics of Belief*. Stanford, CA: CSLI Publications.

World Medical Association. 1964/2008. *Declaration of Helsinki*. Available at http://www.wma.net/en/30publications/10policies/b3/ (accessed March 6, 2009).

Yi, B. Alexander, Oliver Wernet, and Kenneth R. Chien. 2010. "Pregenerative Medicine: Developmental Paradigms in the Biology of Cardiovascular Regeneration," *Journal of Clinical Investigation* 120: 20–8.

Youngner, Stuart. 1988. "Who Defines Futility?" *Journal of the American Medical Association* 260: 2094–5.

Yu, Junying, Kejin Hu, Kim Smuga-Otto, Shulan Tian, et al. 2009. "Human Induced Pluripotent Stem Cells Free of Vector and Transgene Sequences," *Science* 324: 797–801.

Yu, Junying, Maxim A. Vodyanik, Kim Smuga-Otto, Jessica Antosiewicz, et al. 2007. "Induced Pluripotent Stem Cell Lines Derived from Human Somatic Cells," *Science* 318: 1917–20.

Zhao, Tongbiao, Zhen-Ning Zhang, Zhili Rong, and Yang Xu. 2011. "Immunogenicity of Induced Pluripotent Stem Cells," *Nature* 474: 212–15.

Zhao, Xiao-yang, Wei Li, Zhou Lv, Lei Liu, et al. 2009. "iPS Cells Produce Viable Mice through Tetraploid Complementation," *Nature* 461: 86–90.

Zhou, Hongyan, Shili Wu, Jin Young Joo, Saiyong Zhu, et al. 2009. "Generation of Induced Pluripotent Stem Cells Using Recombinant Proteins," *Cell Stem Cell* 4: 381–4.

Zhou, Qiao, Juliana Brown, Andrew Kanarek, Jayaraj Rajagopal, et al. 2008. "In Vivo Reprogramming of Adult Pancreatic Exocrine Cells to Beta-Cells," *Nature* 455: 627–32.

# Index

off-label use, 187, 195, 197–8, 200
oocyte. *See* egg
organs, 21, 109, 114, 164

Parkinson's disease, 41, 43, 46, 156,
    170–4, 176, 179, 193, 199
patients, 2, 9, 12–14, 20, 30, 36, 38, 40–2,
    45–6, 48–51, 55–6, 60, 62, 68, 72–4,
    76, 99, 102, 104, 106, 109, 114–15,
    121, 127, 156–65, 167–79, 182–5, -
    186–201, 202–3
pediatrics, 62, 74, 99, 187
Pegasus, 16–17, 57, 111–12, 129
perfectionism, 6, 64
personhood, 74
persons, 2, 5, 10, 14, 20, 25, 50, 62, 64–5,
    67–9, 72–8, 82, 98, 115, 127, 132–3,
    144, 166, 176, 184
pharmaceutical drugs, 53, 162–3, 168,
    171, 187, 192
Phase I trial, 165, 171–2, 181–2
philosophy, 2, 6–9, 12–13, 18–19, 22,
    27–9, 57–9, 62–3, 65–6, 68–71, 74, 76,
    78–80, 81, 92, 96, 102–3, 107, 121–2,
    126–7, 131–6, 143–4, 146, 148–9,
    151–3, 166, 176, 179–80, 183–4, 203
Pinker, Steven, 137–8
placebo, 173
plasticity, 27, 29–31, 56, 84, 163, 202
postmodernism, 8
potentiality, 10–11, 24
preclinical studies, 15, 49, 56, 110, 161,
    163–8, 186, 194, 196, 198–9, 201
Premack, David and Ann, 139, 144
premodernism, 3, 7, 10–11, 21, 29
privacy, 50–1, 98, 105
properties
    extrinsic properties, 127
    intrinsic properties, 18, 29, 127
    relational properties, 18, 126
propositions, 136–7, 139, 145–6, 148
Proust, Marcel, 1, 186
purity, 51, 53–4, 164

ranking
    cardinal ranking, 178–9, 181
    ordinal ranking, 178–81
Rawls, John, 59
Raz, Joseph, 72, 181–3
Recombinant DNA Advisory Committee
    (RAC), 85, 87
research ethics
    philosophical research ethics, 19
    practical research ethics, 19

research sharing, 94
research subject withdrawl, 97, 175
respect for persons, 69, 72–3, 166
Ricketts, Ed, 114, 140, 152, 203
rights, 2, 6, 8–9, 12, 14, 20, 50–1, 56, 60,
    63, 81, 99–103, 106–7, 132, 202
*Roe v. Wade*, 2
Rousseau, Jean-Jacques, 141–2

Saint Francis, 160
Sartre, Jean-Paul, 177, 181
secular ethics, 10, 14, 60–2, 144
self-consciousness, 126, 135, 143–8,
    150–1, 153
seventeenth century, 3–5, 7, 10, 12,
    56, 202
sham surgery, 170, 173
socialization, 141–2, 150–1
Society of University Surgeons, 194, 200
spinal cord injury, 158, 160–1, 172, 175
Steinbeck, John, 114, 140, 152, 203
Stem Cell Research Oversight Committee,
    87–91, 95–7, 104, 106–7, 123–5
stem cell tourism, 167, 186–9, 191, 195–6,
    199–201
Streiffer, Robert, 110, 116, 130–1

Terrace, Herbert S., 137–8
tetraploid complementation, 32–3, 52
theory of mind, 135, 144–9, 151
therapeutic hope, 158–60, 184–5
therapeutic misconception, 158–9
Thomson, James, 23, 33
tissue banks, 92–3
toxicity, 44, 163–4, 171, 192
transdifferentiation, 24, 33
translational stem cell research, 2, 22, 41,
    58, 101, 110, 121, 200
trial by ordeal, 156–8, 185
tumor, 36, 47, 51, 53, 161, 167, 199
tumorigenicity, 44, 47
Tuskegee Syphilis Study, 75, 81

undue inducement, 94, 104–5
Universal Declaration of Human
    Rights, 127
unnaturalism, 6, 10, 62, 113
utilitarianism, 7, 70
utility, 8, 70, 130, 173, 178

values, 6, 19, 26, 37, 57–9, 63–4, 66, 69,
    72, 75–80, 111, 166, 175–80, 183,
    196, 202
van Leeuwenhoek, Anthony, 4